Frank H. Covey......................................*Words Count:* **91,142**
United States, Nashua, NH, 03063..........*Number of Pages:* **390**
Documented Publishing LLC...................*Book Size:* **5*8 Inches**
documented.publishing@gmail.com

Cortisol
"The Stress Hormone"

Learn About the Master Hormone to Control Your Stress, Anxiety, and Weight.

Frank H. Covey

As a huge thanks for landing on this page, you can enjoy these ***100% FREE Bonuses today!***

• __Bonus 1__

Join Our Exclusive Mastermind
"MEMBERS ONLY"
Group ***for FREE*** Where We Discuss
More About the Book, Share Our Opinions,
and Support Each Other.
Go to: https://bit.ly/Exclusive_Freebies

• __Bonus 2__

Love Audiobooks? Get Instant Access
to The ***Audio Version*** Once Available
For a Limited Time…
Secure Your FREE Copy
Here: bit.ly/Exclusive_Freebies

• __Bonus 3__

Get All Future Updates, Freebies and Offers
Directly with ***NO Extra Charges!***

Legal Notice:

The reader is <u>solely responsible for any actions</u> taken based on the information contained in this book. The author and publisher expressly disclaim any responsibility or liability for any damages or losses incurred by the reader as a result of such actions.

Disclaimer:

This book is intended for <u>educational purposes only.</u> The information contained within is not intended as, and should not be construed as medical, legal, or professional advice. The content is provided as general information and is not a substitute for professional advice or treatment.

__Table of content__

Introduction ____ 9

Chapter 1: How does cortisol affect the body's response to stress? _______________________________ 11

Chapter 2: What are the primary functions of cortisol in the human body? _________________________ 14

Chapter 3: Can cortisol levels be influenced by lifestyle factors such as diet and exercise?______________ 17

Chapter 4: What is the relationship between cortisol and sleep patterns? __________________________ 20

Chapter 5: How does cortisol impact the immune system?______________________________________ 23

Chapter 6: Are there any natural ways to regulate cortisol levels? _______________________________ 26

Chapter 7: Does cortisol play a role in weight management?____________________________________ 29

Chapter 8: Can chronic stress lead to prolonged cortisol elevation?______________________________ 32

Chapter 9: How does cortisol affect memory and cognitive function? _____________________________ 36

Chapter 10: What are the long-term effects of high cortisol levels on overall health? __________________ 40

Chapter 11: Is there a connection between cortisol and anxiety disorders?__________________________ 44

Chapter 12: Can cortisol levels be measured accurately through saliva or blood tests? _________________ 48

Chapter 13: How does cortisol impact the reproductive system in men and women?___________________ 52

Chapter 14: What is the cortisol awakening response and its significance? __________________________ 56

Chapter 15: Can cortisol levels be regulated through mindfulness practices? ________________________ 60

Chapter 16: How does cortisol affect bone health and osteoporosis risk? ___________________________ 64

Chapter 17: What is the role of cortisol in regulating blood sugar levels? ___________________________ 68

Chapter 18: Can cortisol levels be influenced by certain medications?_____________________________ 72

Chapter 19: The Impact of Cortisol on Skin Health and Aging___________________________________ 76

Chapter 20: The Role of Cortisol in the Development and Progression of Cardiovascular Diseases _________ 79

Chapter 21: The Interplay of Cortisol with Other Hormones in the Body ___________________________ 83

Chapter 22: The Relationship between Cortisol and Inflammation________________________________ 87

Chapter 23: The Impact of Environmental Toxins on Cortisol Levels ______________________________ 91

Chapter 24: The Influence of Cortisol on Hair Growth and Loss _________________________________ 95

Chapter 25: The Role of Cortisol in Regulating Blood Pressure __________________________________ 98

Chapter 26: The Influence of Cortisol on the Body's Response to Pain _____________________________ 102

Chapter 27: The Influence of Gut Health and the Microbiome on Cortisol Levels _____________________ 106

Chapter 28: The Effects of Cortisol on the Thyroid Gland and Its Function__________________________ 110

Chapter 29: The Role of Cortisol in the Development and Progression of Autoimmune Diseases___________ 114

Chapter 30: The Influence of Cortisol on the Body's Response to Exercise and Physical Activity ___________ 118

Chapter 31: The Impact of Cortisol on Fertility and Reproductive Health___________________________ 122

Chapter 32: The Impact of Cortisol on the Body's Response to Temperature Regulation _________________ 126

Chapter 33: The Role of Cortisol in Mood Disorders: Depression and Bipolar Disorder__________________ 130

Chapter 34: The Influence of Certain Types of Cancer on Cortisol Levels — 135

Chapter 35: The Fascinating Connection Between Cortisol and the Gut-Brain Axis — 140

Chapter 36: The Influence of Cortisol on Allergies and Allergic Reactions — 145

Chapter 37: The Intriguing Link Between Cortisol and Neurodegenerative Diseases — 150

Chapter 38: The Impact of Chronic Noise and Loud Sounds on Cortisol Levels — 155

Chapter 39: Unraveling the Connection Between Cortisol and Appetite Regulation — 160

Chapter 40: Unveiling the Impact of Cortisol on Vaccinations and Immunizations — 164

Chapter 41: The Intricate Connection Between Cortisol and Metabolic Syndrome — 169

Chapter 42: Unraveling the Relationship Between Cortisol and Hormonal Contraceptives — 174

Chapter 43: Cortisol's Influence on Liver Function and Detoxification Processes — 178

Chapter 44: The Intricate Dance Between Cortisol and Fasting/Calorie Restriction — 182

Chapter 45: Unveiling the Connection Between Cortisol and Gastrointestinal Disorders — 186

Chapter 46: Unraveling the Connection Between Cortisol and Infections — 190

Chapter 47: Unveiling the Complex Relationship Between Cortisol and the Body's Response to Trauma — 193

Chapter 48: The Intricate Dance Between Cortisol and the Body's Response to Environmental Pollutants — 197

Chapter 49: Unraveling the Connection Between Cortisol and Chronic Pain Conditions — 201

Chapter 50: The Sun's Radiance: Exploring the Connection Between Cortisol, Sunlight, and Vitamin D — 204

Chapter 51: Cortisol's Role in the Body's Response to Surgical Procedures: A Journey Towards Healing — 208

Chapter 52: The Intricate Dance Between Cortisol and the Body's Response to Psychological Therapies and Interventions — 212

Chapter 53: The Cortisol Connection: Unveiling the Role of Cortisol in Substance Abuse Disorders — 216

Chapter 54: Unraveling the Genetic Influence on Cortisol Levels: How Genes Shape the Stress Hormone — 219

Chapter 55: Cortisol and Acute Injuries: Understanding the Body's Response to Recovery — 222

Chapter 56: Navigating the Hormonal Journey: Cortisol's Influence on Pregnancy and Maternal Well-being — 225

Chapter 57: Unraveling the Complex Connection: Cortisol's Role in Eating Disorders — 229

Chapter 58: Unraveling the Electromagnetic Connection: Exploring the Influence of Electromagnetic Fields on Cortisol Levels — 232

Chapter 59: Embracing the Elements: Cortisol's Influence on the Body's Response to Heat and Cold Stress — 236

Chapter 60: Navigating the Medication Maze: Cortisol's Influence on the Body's Response and Drug Interactions — 240

Chapter 61: Breathing Under the Influence: Exploring Cortisol's Impact on the Development and Progression of Lung Diseases — 244

Chapter 62: The Social Hormone: Exploring the Influence of Social Interactions and Support Networks on Cortisol Levels — 248

Chapter 63: The Cortisol-Allergic Asthma Connection: Unveiling the Body's Response to Respiratory Allergies — 252

Chapter 64: Unveiling the Cortisol-Pollutant Connection: Exploring the Impact of Environmental Pollutants on the Body's Stress Response — 256

Chapter 65: The Cortisol-Kidney Connection: Exploring the Impact of Cortisol on Kidney Health — 260

Chapter 66: The Cortisol-Air Pollution Connection: Exploring the Impact of Air Pollution and Smog on Cortisol Levels — 264

Chapter 67: Cortisol and Radiation Exposure: Understanding the Body's Response — 268

Chapter 68: Navigating Menopause: Exploring the Influence of Cortisol on Hormonal Changes — 271

Chapter 69: Unveiling the Connection Between Cortisol and Liver Diseases _______________________ 275

Chapter 70: Unveiling the Impact of Heavy Metals and Toxins on Cortisol Levels _______________________ 278

Chapter 71: Unraveling the Connection Between Cortisol and Autoimmune Hepatitis _______________________ 281

Chapter 72: Unveiling the Impact of Cortisol on the Body's Response to Psychological Trauma _______________________ 285

Chapter 73: Unveiling the Role of Cortisol in Heart Failure _______________________ 289

Chapter 74: Shedding Light on the Influence of Pesticides and Insecticides on Cortisol Levels _______________________ 292

Chapter 75: Unraveling the Impact of Cortisol on the Body's Response to Chemotherapy _______________________ 295

Chapter 76: Navigating the Impact of Cortisol on the Body's Response to Hormonal Changes During Puberty _______________________ 298

Chapter 77: Understanding the Role of Cortisol in the Development and Progression of Rheumatoid Arthritis _______________________ 301

Chapter 78: Understanding the Potential Influence of Electromagnetic Radiation on Cortisol Levels _______________________ 305

Chapter 79: Unraveling the Relationship Between Cortisol and the Body's Response to Chronic Fatigue Syndrome _______________________ 309

Chapter 80: Unraveling the Impact of Cortisol on the Body's Response to Chronic Pain Conditions _______________________ 313

Chapter 81: Unraveling the Role of Cortisol in the Development and Progression of Multiple Sclerosis _______________________ 317

Chapter 82: Unraveling the Influence of Industrial Chemicals and Solvents on Cortisol Levels _______________________ 320

Chapter 83: Unveiling the Impact of Cortisol on the Body's Response to Organ Transplantation _______________________ 324

Chapter 84: The Intricate Dance of Cortisol and Hormonal Changes During the Menstrual Cycle _______________________ 328

Chapter 85: Exploring the Connection Between Cortisol and Crohn's Disease _______________________ 332

Chapter 86: Unraveling the Impact of Endocrine-Disrupting Chemicals on Cortisol Levels _______________________ 336

Chapter 87: Understanding the Connection Between Cortisol and Post-Traumatic Stress Disorder (PTSD) _______________________ 340

Chapter 88: Unraveling the Impact of Cortisol on the Body's Response to Chronic Kidney Disease _______________________ 344

Chapter 89: Unveiling the Relationship Between Cortisol and Parkinson's Disease _______________________ 348

Chapter 90: Unveiling the Impact of Noise Pollution and Traffic Noise on Cortisol Levels _______________________ 352

Chapter 91: Unraveling the Influence of Cortisol on the Body's Response to Organ Rejection after Transplantation _______________________ 355

Chapter 92: Unraveling the Impact of Cortisol on the Body's Response to Hormonal Changes during the Aging Process _______________________ 358

Chapter 93: Unraveling the Role of Cortisol in the Development and Progression of Ulcerative Colitis _______________________ 362

Chapter 94: Unveiling the Impact of Household Chemicals and Cleaning Products on Cortisol Levels _______________________ 366

Chapter 95: Unveiling the Link Between Cortisol and the Body's Response to Obsessive-Compulsive Disorder (OCD) _______________________ 369

Chapter 96: Unveiling the Impact of Cortisol on the Body's Response to Chronic Obstructive Pulmonary Disease (COPD) _______________________ 372

Chapter 97: The Intriguing Connection Between Cortisol and Amyotrophic Lateral Sclerosis (ALS) _______________________ 376

Chapter 98: Unveiling the Impact of Indoor Air Pollutants and Mold on Cortisol Levels _______________________ 380

Chapter 99: Unraveling the Impact of Cortisol on the Body's Response to Organ Failure and Transplantation _______________________ 384

So, _______________________ 388

Introduction

Welcome to the captivating world of cortisol, a hormone that plays a pivotal role in our bodies' response to stress and influences various aspects of our health and well-being. In this book, we embark on an exploratory journey through unique chapters, each shedding light on a different facet of cortisol's impact on our lives. From its effects on the body's stress response to its role in various diseases and conditions, we dive deep into the fascinating world of cortisol and its intricate connections to our physical and mental well-being.

Chapter by chapter, we uncover the profound influence of cortisol on different body systems and functions. We unravel the relationship between cortisol and stress, investigating how this hormone affects our body's response to challenging situations and influences our ability to adapt and cope. We explore the connections between cortisol and sleep, immune function, memory, weight management, and the reproductive system, among many other captivating topics.

We delve into the complex interplay between cortisol and various health conditions, examining its involvement in anxiety disorders, depression, autoimmune diseases, and even neurodegenerative disorders. We explore how cortisol levels can be influenced by lifestyle factors, medications, environmental exposures, and genetic predispositions, unveiling the intricate web of factors that contribute to cortisol regulation.

Whether you are a healthcare professional, a student of biology or psychology, or simply someone interested in understanding the intricate workings of the human body, this book is for you.

We invite you to embark on this enlightening journey as we unravel the mysteries of cortisol. Prepare to be captivated by the intricate connections between this remarkable hormone and our physical and emotional well-being. Whether you're seeking knowledge, practical insights, or simply a deeper understanding of the fascinating world of hormones, this book promises to be an invaluable resource.

So, turn the page, dive into the chapters, and let us explore the intricate tapestry of cortisol together. Let's unlock the secrets of this remarkable hormone and discover how it shapes our lives in ways we never imagined.

Chapter 1: How does cortisol affect the body's response to stress?

In this chapter, we will dive into the fascinating world of cortisol and explore its intricate relationship with stress. Stress is an inevitable part of life, and our bodies have evolved intricate mechanisms to deal with it. One of the key players in our stress response is cortisol, a hormone produced by the adrenal glands. But how does cortisol really affect our body's response to stress? Let's embark on this journey to unravel the secrets of cortisol and its impact on our well-being.

Understanding Stress:

Before we delve into the role of cortisol, it's crucial to understand what stress is. Stress can be triggered by various factors, such as demanding workloads, relationship difficulties, or financial pressures. When we encounter a stressful situation, our bodies initiate a complex response known as the "fight-or-flight" response. This response prepares us to face or escape from potential threats by releasing a cascade of hormones, including cortisol.

The Role of Cortisol:

Cortisol is often referred to as the "stress hormone" because it plays a pivotal role in the stress response. It helps regulate a wide range of bodily functions, including metabolism, immune response, blood pressure, and the body's inflammatory processes. Cortisol is released in response to signals from the brain's hypothalamus and pituitary gland, which detect stress and activate the adrenal glands to produce and release cortisol into the bloodstream.

Immediate Effects of Cortisol:

When cortisol is released into the bloodstream, it quickly travels to various parts of the body, ready to mobilize energy and resources for the imminent stressor. In the short term, cortisol helps increase blood sugar levels, providing a quick burst of energy to cope with the demands of the situation. It also enhances cardiovascular function, improving oxygen delivery to muscles and sharpening our focus and attention.

Long-term Effects of Cortisol:

While cortisol's immediate effects are beneficial for coping with acute stress, prolonged or chronic stress can lead to persistently elevated cortisol levels. This continuous exposure to high cortisol levels can have detrimental effects on our physical and mental health. Chronic elevation of cortisol has been associated with conditions such as hypertension, impaired immune function, increased abdominal fat deposition, and even cognitive impairment.

Cortisol and the Immune System:

Another critical aspect of cortisol's role in stress response is its impact on the immune system. In the short term, cortisol suppresses certain immune responses, which helps divert resources to address the immediate threat. However, chronic elevation of cortisol can weaken the immune system, making us more susceptible to infections, inflammatory diseases, and slower wound healing.

Cortisol and Mood:

Beyond its physiological effects, cortisol also influences our emotional and mental well-being. Prolonged stress and elevated cortisol levels have been linked to mood disorders, such as depression and anxiety. Cortisol can affect neurotransmitter levels in the brain, altering our mood, sleep patterns, and overall emotional balance.

Regulating Cortisol Levels:

Given the potential negative consequences of chronically elevated cortisol, it becomes crucial to find ways to regulate its levels. Fortunately, there are several strategies that can help manage cortisol levels effectively. Regular exercise, adequate sleep, stress management techniques like meditation and deep breathing, and engaging in activities we enjoy can all contribute to maintaining cortisol within a healthy range.

So,

Cortisol is a remarkable hormone that plays a vital role in our body's response to stress. While it helps us cope with immediate challenges, prolonged elevation of cortisol levels can have significant implications for our physical and mental well-being. Understanding the impact of cortisol on our body can empower us to take proactive steps to manage stress, optimize our health, and promote a balanced lifestyle. By adopting healthy habits and seeking support when needed, we can navigate the intricate dance between cortisol and stress, paving the way for a happier, healthier life.

Chapter 2: What are the primary functions of cortisol in the human body?

We will embark on an exciting exploration of the primary functions of cortisol in the human body. Cortisol, often known as the "stress hormone," is a fascinating molecule with a wide range of essential roles beyond its association with stress. In this chapter, we will uncover the hidden depths of cortisol and discover how it influences our body's intricate systems in ways that go far beyond our initial expectations.

Cortisol's Role in Metabolism:

One of the central functions of cortisol is its role in regulating metabolism. Cortisol acts as a metabolic controller, influencing various aspects of energy utilization and storage. It stimulates gluconeogenesis, a process where the liver produces glucose from non-carbohydrate sources, such as amino acids, to maintain adequate blood sugar levels. This ensures a steady supply of energy during fasting or periods of stress.

Additionally, cortisol facilitates the breakdown of stored glycogen in the liver and muscles, releasing glucose into the bloodstream for immediate energy needs. It also promotes the breakdown of fats and proteins, providing alternative sources of fuel for the body. These metabolic actions of cortisol help sustain energy availability during times of increased demand.

Cortisol and Inflammation:

Another crucial role of cortisol is its influence on the body's inflammatory response. Inflammation is a natural defense mechanism against injury and infection. However, an excessive or prolonged inflammatory response can lead to tissue damage and chronic diseases. Cortisol acts as a potent anti-inflammatory agent by suppressing the immune system's inflammatory processes.

When an inflammatory response is initiated, cortisol inhibits the production of pro-inflammatory substances, such as cytokines and prostaglandins. It also reduces the migration of immune cells to sites of inflammation, dampening the overall inflammatory cascade. This anti-inflammatory effect is vital for maintaining a balanced immune response and preventing excessive tissue damage.

Cortisol's Impact on the Immune System:

Beyond its anti-inflammatory effects, cortisol plays a broader role in modulating the immune system. It influences the function of various immune cells, including lymphocytes, monocytes, and natural killer cells. Cortisol can suppress immune cell proliferation, cytokine production, and antibody synthesis.

While this immunosuppressive effect of cortisol can be beneficial in certain situations, prolonged or excessive cortisol levels can weaken the immune system's ability to defend against pathogens. Individuals with chronically elevated cortisol levels may be more susceptible to infections and experience slower wound healing. Striking a balance between cortisol's immunosuppressive actions and immune system function is crucial for overall health and well-being.

Cortisol and Stress Response:

As we briefly mentioned earlier, cortisol plays a pivotal role in the body's response to stress. When confronted with a stressful situation, the brain's hypothalamus releases corticotropin-releasing hormone (CRH), which signals the pituitary gland to secrete adrenocorticotropic hormone (ACTH). ACTH then stimulates the adrenal glands to release cortisol into the bloodstream.

This surge in cortisol prepares the body for the challenges of the stressor. It enhances cardiovascular function, increases blood sugar levels, and sharpens focus and attention. These immediate responses help us respond effectively to the stressor at hand. However, chronic stress and persistently elevated cortisol levels can have detrimental effects on various bodily systems, as we explored in Chapter 1.

Cortisol and Sleep-Wake Cycle:

In addition to its roles in metabolism, inflammation, immune function, and stress response, cortisol also influences our sleep-wake cycle. Cortisol levels follow a diurnal pattern, with the highest levels in the morning upon awakening and gradually decreasing throughout the day. This pattern helps us wake up feeling refreshed and alert, ready to face the challenges of the day.

Cortisol's interaction with the sleep-wake cycle is intricate. Elevated cortisol levels in the evening can interfere with the onset of sleep and disrupt the quality of sleep. Inadequate sleep, in turn, can impact cortisol regulation, leading to a vicious cycle of sleep disruption and dysregulated cortisol levels. Maintaining a healthy sleep routine and practicing relaxation techniques before bedtime can help optimize cortisol levels and promote restful sleep.

So,

Cortisol, often referred to as the "stress hormone," has far-reaching effects beyond its association with stress. Its primary functions encompass metabolism regulation, modulation of the inflammatory response, influence on the immune system, orchestration of the stress response, and involvement in the sleep-wake cycle. Cortisol is an intricate player in the symphony of our body's systems, ensuring energy availability, balancing inflammation, and fine-tuning our immune response.

Understanding the multifaceted functions of cortisol provides us with a greater appreciation for its significance in maintaining overall health and well-being. By adopting stress-management techniques, promoting a healthy sleep routine, and cultivating a balanced lifestyle, we can optimize cortisol's actions in our body and foster a harmonious interplay between this vital hormone and our intricate physiological processes.

Chapter 3: Can cortisol levels be influenced by lifestyle factors such as diet and exercise?

We will explore the intriguing connection between cortisol levels and lifestyle factors such as diet and exercise. Cortisol, the "stress hormone," plays a crucial role in our body's response to stress. However, it's important to understand that cortisol levels can also be influenced by various aspects of our lifestyle. In this chapter, we will delve into the fascinating relationship between cortisol and lifestyle choices, shedding light on how diet and exercise can impact our cortisol levels.

The Link Between Cortisol and Diet:

Our dietary choices can have a significant impact on cortisol levels. Certain foods and nutrients can either promote or mitigate cortisol release in response to stress. Let's explore some key factors that can influence cortisol levels through diet:

Nutrient Balance:

Maintaining a well-balanced diet with adequate intake of macronutrients (carbohydrates, proteins, and fats) is important for cortisol regulation. Low-carbohydrate diets, for example, can increase cortisol levels due to the body's increased reliance on alternative fuel sources. On the other hand, consuming a balanced diet that includes healthy carbohydrates, proteins, and fats can help stabilize cortisol levels.

Caffeine and Stimulants:

Beverages containing caffeine, such as coffee and energy drinks, can temporarily elevate cortisol levels. While moderate caffeine consumption may not pose significant issues for most individuals, excessive intake or sensitivity to caffeine can lead to chronically elevated cortisol levels. It's advisable to moderate caffeine consumption, especially if you are sensitive to its effects.

Sugar and Processed Foods:

High sugar and processed food diets have been associated with dysregulation of cortisol levels. Consuming excessive amounts of refined sugar and processed foods can lead to spikes and crashes in blood sugar levels, triggering the release of cortisol to maintain glucose balance. Opting for whole foods, complex carbohydrates, and a balanced intake of macronutrients can help stabilize cortisol levels.

Micronutrients:

Certain micronutrients, such as vitamin C, vitamin B5, and magnesium, play important roles in cortisol regulation. Including a variety of nutrient-dense foods in your diet, such as fruits, vegetables, whole grains, nuts, and seeds, can help ensure an adequate intake of these micronutrients, supporting healthy cortisol levels.

Exercise and Cortisol Regulation:

Physical activity and exercise also play a significant role in cortisol regulation. While exercise temporarily elevates cortisol levels, regular physical activity has a positive impact on cortisol regulation in the long term. Let's explore how exercise influences cortisol levels:

Acute Exercise:

Engaging in intense or prolonged exercise can lead to a temporary increase in cortisol levels. This cortisol response is a natural part of the body's adaptation to the physical stress placed on it during exercise. However, this acute increase in cortisol is usually short-lived and is followed by a subsequent decrease as the body recovers.

Regular Exercise:

Consistent participation in exercise has been shown to improve cortisol regulation. Regular exercise helps the body adapt to stress more effectively, reducing the overall cortisol response. It promotes a healthy stress response system and helps restore cortisol levels to baseline more efficiently after a stressful event.

Exercise Type and Intensity:

The type and intensity of exercise can influence cortisol levels differently. Moderate-intensity aerobic exercises, such as brisk walking, jogging, or cycling, have been shown to have positive effects on cortisol regulation. High-intensity interval training (HIIT) and resistance training can also be beneficial. However, prolonged, intense exercise without adequate recovery periods may lead to chronically elevated cortisol levels.

Mind-Body Exercises:

Mind-body exercises like yoga, tai chi, and meditation have gained attention for their potential to reduce cortisol levels. These practices incorporate relaxation techniques, deep breathing, and mindfulness, which help activate the body's relaxation response and counteract the effects of stress on cortisol regulation.

So,

Diet and exercise are powerful lifestyle factors that can influence cortisol levels. While diet choices can impact cortisol through nutrient balance, caffeine and stimulant intake, sugar and processed foods, and the consumption of essential micronutrients, exercise plays a dynamic role in acute and chronic cortisol regulation. Regular exercise, especially moderate-intensity aerobic activities, promotes a healthy stress response and aids in cortisol regulation.

By making mindful choices in our diet, emphasizing whole foods, and avoiding excessive caffeine and processed foods, we can support healthy cortisol levels. Incorporating regular physical activity, including a mix of aerobic exercises, resistance training, and mind-body practices, can help us effectively manage cortisol and optimize our stress response. Striving for a balanced lifestyle that nourishes our body and mind sets the stage for a harmonious relationship between cortisol and our overall well-being.

Chapter 4: What is the relationship between cortisol and sleep patterns?

We will explore the fascinating relationship between cortisol and sleep patterns. Sleep is a fundamental aspect of our well-being, and cortisol, the "stress hormone," plays a significant role in regulating our sleep-wake cycle. In this chapter, we will delve into the intricate connection between cortisol and sleep, shedding light on how cortisol levels can affect our ability to fall asleep, stay asleep, and wake up feeling refreshed.

The Circadian Rhythm and Cortisol:

To understand the relationship between cortisol and sleep patterns, it's crucial to grasp the concept of the circadian rhythm. Our bodies have an internal biological clock that regulates various physiological processes, including the sleep-wake cycle. Cortisol follows a diurnal pattern, with its highest levels upon awakening and gradually decreasing throughout the day.

In the early morning hours, the hypothalamus releases corticotropin-releasing hormone (CRH), which signals the pituitary gland to secrete adrenocorticotropic hormone (ACTH). ACTH, in turn, stimulates the adrenal glands to release cortisol into the bloodstream, helping us wake up and feel alert. As the day progresses, cortisol levels gradually decline, reaching their lowest point in the evening, preparing the body for restorative sleep.

Cortisol and Falling Asleep:

Optimal cortisol regulation is crucial for our ability to fall asleep. When cortisol levels are elevated in the evening, it can interfere with the onset of sleep. Stressful events or chronic stress can lead to heightened cortisol release, making it difficult to unwind and relax before bedtime. Additionally, exposure to bright light, especially blue light emitted by electronic devices, can suppress the release of melatonin, the hormone that helps regulate sleep-wake cycles. This, in turn, can disrupt the normal decline in cortisol levels, leading to delayed sleep onset. Creating a soothing bedtime routine, minimizing exposure to stimulating activities and bright lights, and establishing a sleep-friendly environment can help regulate cortisol levels and promote a smoother transition into sleep.

Cortisol and Sleep Maintenance:

In addition to falling asleep, cortisol levels can also impact our ability to maintain sleep throughout the night. Cortisol acts as a natural stimulant, preparing the body for action and vigilance. When cortisol levels remain elevated during sleep, it can increase alertness, making it harder to stay asleep and increasing the likelihood of sleep disturbances.

Chronic elevation of cortisol levels due to ongoing stress or other factors can disrupt the normal sleep architecture, leading to fragmented sleep and frequent awakenings. These awakenings may not always be consciously noticed but can still impact the overall quality of sleep. Managing stress, adopting relaxation techniques before bedtime, and creating a sleep-friendly environment can help mitigate the impact of elevated cortisol on sleep maintenance.

Cortisol and Morning Awakening:

As cortisol follows a diurnal pattern, it reaches its peak levels in the morning, helping us wake up and feel alert. This surge in cortisol is part of the body's natural awakening response, ensuring we have the necessary energy and focus to start our day. However, individuals with irregular cortisol patterns or those experiencing chronic stress may have disruptions in this awakening response.

Some individuals may experience a delayed peak in cortisol levels, leading to difficulties in waking up and feeling groggy in the morning. Others may have an exaggerated cortisol response upon awakening, resulting in a sudden spike in alertness. These variations in cortisol patterns can affect the overall quality of morning awakening and contribute to feelings of fatigue or sluggishness throughout the day.

Regulating Cortisol for Better Sleep:

Managing cortisol levels is crucial for optimizing sleep patterns. Here are some strategies to help regulate cortisol and promote better sleep:

Establish a Consistent Sleep Schedule: Maintaining a regular sleep schedule, including consistent bedtimes and wake-up times, helps regulate cortisol patterns and reinforces the body's natural circadian rhythm.

Create a Relaxing Bedtime Routine: Engaging in relaxing activities before bed, such as reading, taking a warm bath, or practicing relaxation techniques like deep breathing or meditation, can help lower cortisol levels and prepare the body for sleep.

Minimize Stimulating Activities: Limit exposure to electronic devices, bright lights, and stimulating activities close to bedtime, as they can interfere with melatonin production and disrupt the normal decline in cortisol levels.

Promote a Sleep-Friendly Environment: Create a cool, dark, and quiet sleep environment that promotes relaxation and minimizes disruptions. Consider using blackout curtains, earplugs, or white noise machines to enhance sleep quality.

Manage Stress: Adopt stress-management techniques such as exercise, mindfulness practices, and engaging in activities that promote relaxation and well-being. Managing stress helps regulate cortisol levels and supports healthy sleep patterns.

So,

Cortisol and sleep patterns share an intricate relationship. Optimal cortisol regulation is essential for falling asleep, maintaining sleep, and experiencing a refreshing awakening in the morning. Disruptions in cortisol levels, whether due to stress, irregular sleep schedules, or exposure to stimulating factors, can impact the quality and quantity of sleep.

By adopting healthy sleep habits, managing stress, and creating a sleep-friendly environment, we can support the regulation of cortisol and promote better sleep. Striving for a balance between cortisol's awakening response and its decline throughout the day sets the stage for a harmonious relationship between cortisol and our sleep-wake cycle, leading to more restful nights and rejuvenating mornings.

Chapter 5: How does cortisol impact the immune system?

We will explore the intricate relationship between cortisol and the immune system. Cortisol, known as the "stress hormone," plays a crucial role in our body's response to stress. However, its influence extends beyond the stress response and into our immune system. In this chapter, we will delve into the fascinating ways in which cortisol impacts the immune system, shedding light on its dual role as both a regulator and modulator of immune function.

The Immune System: A Balancing Act:

The immune system is our body's defense mechanism against pathogens, infections, and other harmful invaders. It comprises a complex network of cells, tissues, and organs working together to protect our health. However, maintaining a balanced immune response is crucial, as an overactive immune system can lead to autoimmune diseases, while an underactive immune system can make us susceptible to infections and diseases.

Cortisol's Anti-Inflammatory Effects:

One of the keyways in which cortisol impacts the immune system is through its anti-inflammatory effects. When the immune system is activated in response to an injury or infection, it releases pro-inflammatory substances called cytokines. While inflammation is a natural part of the immune response, excessive or prolonged inflammation can lead to tissue damage and chronic diseases.

Cortisol acts as a potent anti-inflammatory agent by inhibiting the production of pro-inflammatory cytokines and other immune signaling molecules. It helps regulate the intensity and duration of the immune response, preventing excessive inflammation. This anti-inflammatory effect of cortisol is crucial for maintaining a balanced immune system and preventing chronic inflammation-related conditions.

Immunosuppressive Effects of Cortisol:

In addition to its anti-inflammatory effects, cortisol also has immunosuppressive properties. Prolonged exposure to high levels of cortisol can suppress certain aspects of immune function, including the proliferation and activity of immune cells. This is part of the body's mechanism to conserve energy and resources during times of stress or injury.

Cortisol can inhibit the production and function of various immune cells, such as lymphocytes and monocytes, as well as the production of antibodies. It can also dampen the immune response to vaccines and impair the body's ability to mount an effective defense against pathogens. While these immunosuppressive effects are beneficial in the short term to divert resources to address immediate threats, chronically elevated cortisol levels can weaken the immune system's ability to fight infections and maintain optimal health.

Stress, Cortisol, and Immune Function:

Stress has a profound impact on our immune system, and cortisol plays a central role in mediating this interaction. During times of stress, the brain's hypothalamus releases corticotropin-releasing hormone (CRH), which signals the pituitary gland to secrete adrenocorticotropic hormone (ACTH). ACTH then stimulates the adrenal glands to produce and release cortisol into the bloodstream.

While cortisol helps mobilize energy and resources for the stress response, chronic stress and persistently elevated cortisol levels can have detrimental effects on immune function. High cortisol levels can impair the immune system's ability to fight infections, increase susceptibility to viral and bacterial illnesses, and slow down wound healing.

It's worth noting that the impact of stress and cortisol on the immune system can vary among individuals. Factors such as genetics, age, overall health, and duration of stress can influence the extent to which cortisol affects immune function. Additionally, individual differences in cortisol sensitivity and immune response contribute to variations in the body's immune reactions to stress.

Balancing Cortisol and Immune Function:

Maintaining a balanced cortisol level is crucial for optimal immune function. While cortisol has both anti-inflammatory and immunosuppressive effects, chronic elevation of cortisol levels can compromise immune system function. Striking a balance between cortisol regulation and immune response is essential for overall health and well-being.

Here are some strategies to help support a balanced immune system and cortisol regulation:

Stress Management:

Effective stress management techniques, such as mindfulness practices, deep breathing exercises, and engaging in activities that promote relaxation, can help lower cortisol levels, and reduce the impact of chronic stress on immune function.

Regular Exercise:

Regular physical activity has been shown to have immune-modulating effects and help regulate cortisol levels. Aim for moderate-intensity aerobic exercises, such as brisk walking or cycling, as well as activities that promote strength and flexibility.

Healthy Lifestyle Choices:

Adopting a healthy lifestyle that includes a balanced diet, adequate sleep, and avoiding excessive ... and tobacco use can help support a balanced immune system and cortisol regulation.

Social Support:

Maintaining strong social connections and seeking support from loved ones can help buffer the impact of stress on cortisol levels and immune function.

So,

Cortisol's impact on the immune system is multifaceted, with both anti-inflammatory and immunosuppressive effects. While cortisol helps regulate the intensity and duration of immune responses, chronic elevation of cortisol levels can compromise immune function. Striking a balance between cortisol regulation and immune response is crucial for maintaining a healthy immune system.

By adopting stress management techniques, engaging in regular exercise, making healthy lifestyle choices, and fostering social connections, we can support a balanced immune system and cortisol regulation. This, in turn, promotes overall health, resilience, and the body's ability to mount an effective immune response when faced with challenges.

Chapter 6: Are there any natural ways to regulate cortisol levels?

We will explore natural ways to regulate cortisol levels. Cortisol, the "stress hormone," plays a crucial role in our body's response to stress. However, chronic elevation of cortisol levels can have negative implications for our health and well-being. In this chapter, we will delve into the fascinating realm of natural approaches that can help regulate cortisol levels, promoting balance and overall wellness in our lives.

Stress Management Techniques:

One of the most effective ways to regulate cortisol levels is through stress management techniques. Chronic stress is a significant contributor to elevated cortisol levels. By incorporating stress-reducing practices into our daily lives, we can help lower cortisol and create a more balanced state of being. Some effective stress management techniques include:

• Mindfulness Meditation: Practicing mindfulness meditation involves focusing on the present moment and cultivating an attitude of non-judgmental awareness. Research suggests that regular mindfulness meditation can help reduce cortisol levels and promote relaxation.

• Deep Breathing Exercises: Deep breathing exercises, such as diaphragmatic breathing or box breathing, can activate the body's relaxation response. By slowing down our breath and taking deep, deliberate inhalations and exhalations, we can help regulate cortisol and induce a state of calm.

• Yoga and Tai Chi: These mind-body practices combine movement, breath control, and meditation. Engaging in yoga or tai chi can help reduce stress and regulate cortisol levels. These practices emphasize physical and mental well-being, promoting relaxation and inner balance.

Regular Physical Activity:

Exercise is a natural cortisol regulator, promoting overall physical and mental well-being. Engaging in regular physical activity helps burn off excess cortisol and releases endorphins, the body's natural mood-enhancing chemicals. Here are some key points to consider:

• Moderate-Intensity Aerobic Exercise: Activities like brisk walking, jogging, swimming, or cycling can help regulate cortisol levels. Aim for at least 150 minutes of moderate-intensity aerobic exercise per week, or as recommended by your healthcare professional.

• Strength Training: Incorporating strength training exercises, such as weightlifting or resistance training, into your fitness routine can also help regulate cortisol. Strength training improves muscle mass, increases metabolism, and promotes overall hormonal balance.

• Mind-Body Exercises: Mind-body practices like yoga, Pilates, and qigong integrate physical movement with breath control and mental focus. These exercises can have a calming effect on the body and mind, reducing cortisol levels and promoting relaxation.

Adequate Sleep:

Sleep plays a vital role in cortisol regulation. Chronic sleep deprivation or poor sleep quality can contribute to elevated cortisol levels. Prioritize healthy sleep habits to support optimal cortisol regulation:

• Consistent Sleep Schedule: Aim for a regular sleep schedule, going to bed and waking up at the same time each day, even on weekends. This consistency helps regulate the body's natural circadian rhythm and cortisol patterns.

• Create a Sleep-Friendly Environment: Ensure your bedroom is cool, dark, and quiet. Consider using blackout curtains, earplugs, or white noise machines to create an ideal sleep environment.

• Establish a Relaxing Bedtime Routine: Engage in calming activities before bed, such as reading a book, taking a warm bath, or practicing relaxation techniques like deep breathing or meditation. These rituals signal the body that it's time to wind down and promote restful sleep.

Healthy Diet and Nutrition:

What we eat can also impact cortisol levels. A healthy, balanced diet can help regulate cortisol and support overall well-being. Consider the following nutritional strategies:

• Balanced Macronutrient Intake: Include a mix of carbohydrates, proteins, and healthy fats in your meals. Avoid extremely low-carbohydrate diets, as they may increase cortisol levels.
• Limit Caffeine Intake: Excessive caffeine consumption can elevate cortisol levels. Limit your intake of coffee, tea, energy drinks, and other caffeinated beverages, especially in the afternoon and evening.
• Avoid Excessive Sugar and Processed Foods: High sugar and processed food diets can contribute to dysregulated cortisol levels. Opt for whole, unprocessed foods and prioritize nutrient-dense choices.
• Incorporate Stress-Reducing Foods: Some foods have natural stress-reducing properties. Consider incorporating foods rich in omega-3 fatty acids (e.g., fatty fish, flaxseeds), antioxidants (e.g., berries, dark leafy greens), and magnesium (e.g., spinach, almonds) into your diet.

Social Support and Relaxation:

Maintaining social connections and engaging in activities that promote relaxation are important for cortisol regulation. Spending quality time with loved ones, participating in hobbies or creative pursuits, and engaging in activities that bring joy and relaxation can all contribute to a sense of well-being and help reduce cortisol levels.

So,

Regulating cortisol levels is essential for overall health and well-being. By adopting natural approaches to manage stress, engaging in regular physical activity, prioritizing adequate sleep, maintaining a healthy diet, and fostering social connections, we can support cortisol regulation and promote balance in our lives.

Remember, each person is unique, and finding the right combination of strategies that work for you is important. Experiment with different techniques, be patient with yourself, and listen to your body. By incorporating these natural approaches into your lifestyle, you can take positive steps towards regulating cortisol and cultivating a healthier, more balanced life.

Chapter 7: Does cortisol play a role in weight management?

We will explore the intriguing relationship between cortisol and weight management. Cortisol, known as the "stress hormone," is involved in various physiological processes in the body. One area of interest is its potential impact on weight regulation. In this chapter, we will delve into the role cortisol plays in weight management, shedding light on how cortisol levels can influence body weight and the interplay between stress, cortisol, and our relationship with food.

Understanding Cortisol and Weight:

Before we dive into the specifics, it's important to understand the basics of weight management. Body weight is influenced by a complex interplay of factors, including genetics, metabolism, physical activity, and dietary choices. Cortisol, as a hormone involved in stress response and metabolism, has been studied for its potential involvement in weight regulation.

Cortisol and Abdominal Fat:

One area of focus in cortisol research is its relationship with abdominal fat deposition. Excess weight carried around the abdomen, often referred to as visceral or central adiposity, is associated with an increased risk of metabolic disorders, such as type 2 diabetes and cardiovascular disease.

Studies have suggested that chronic exposure to elevated cortisol levels may contribute to abdominal fat accumulation. Cortisol promotes the breakdown of stored glycogen in the liver, leading to increased blood glucose levels. In response, the body releases insulin to manage the glucose, and elevated insulin levels can promote the storage of excess calories as fat, particularly in the abdominal region.

Cortisol, Stress, and Emotional Eating:

Another aspect of the cortisol-weight relationship revolves around stress and emotional eating. When we experience stress, cortisol levels rise, triggering physiological changes to help us cope with the perceived threat. One common response to stress is an increase in appetite, particularly for calorie-dense, highly palatable foods.

In times of stress, cortisol can stimulate cravings for comfort foods that are often high in sugar, fat, and salt. Consuming these foods may temporarily provide a sense of comfort and pleasure, but over time, they can contribute to weight gain. Additionally, chronic stress and elevated cortisol levels can disrupt hunger and satiety signals, leading to overeating and difficulty in regulating food intake.

Cortisol and Metabolism:

Cortisol also plays a role in metabolic regulation, influencing energy expenditure and nutrient utilization. In response to stress, cortisol increases blood sugar levels, providing a quick energy source for the body to cope with the perceived threat. This can lead to an increase in appetite and cravings for energy-dense foods.

However, chronically elevated cortisol levels can have implications for metabolism. Prolonged exposure to high cortisol levels can affect insulin sensitivity, impair glucose utilization, and promote the breakdown of muscle proteins. These metabolic changes can contribute to weight gain and hinder weight loss efforts.

Strategies for Managing Cortisol and Weight:

While cortisol's impact on weight management is complex, there are strategies that can help support a healthy balance:

Stress Management:

Effective stress management techniques can help regulate cortisol levels and minimize the impact of chronic stress on weight. Engage in activities such as mindfulness meditation, deep breathing exercises, yoga, or engaging hobbies that promote relaxation and reduce stress.

Regular Physical Activity:

Exercise plays a vital role in weight management and cortisol regulation. Engage in regular physical activity, combining cardiovascular exercises with strength training, as it helps burn calories, reduces stress, and promotes overall well-being.

Adequate Sleep:

Prioritize quality sleep as insufficient or poor-quality sleep can lead to increased cortisol levels and disrupt metabolic processes. Aim for a consistent sleep schedule, create a relaxing sleep environment, and establish a bedtime routine that promotes restful sleep.

Balanced Diet:

Adopting a balanced diet that includes whole, nutrient-dense foods can help regulate cortisol levels and support weight management. Include a mix of lean proteins, whole grains, fruits, vegetables, and healthy fats in your meals. Avoid restrictive diets or severe calorie restrictions, as they can elevate cortisol and disrupt metabolic processes.

Mindful Eating:

Practicing mindful eating can help break the cycle of stress-driven overeating. Pay attention to physical hunger and fullness cues, eat slowly, and savor each bite. Cultivate a balanced and positive relationship with food, focusing on nourishing the body rather than using it as a coping mechanism for stress.

Social Support:

Maintaining social connections and seeking support from loved ones can help buffer the impact of stress on cortisol levels and weight management. Share your journey with trusted individuals who can provide encouragement and support.

So,

While cortisol's role in weight management is complex, it does play a role in certain aspects of body weight regulation. Chronic exposure to elevated cortisol levels, particularly in the context of stress, can contribute to abdominal fat accumulation and affect metabolic processes related to weight management.

By implementing strategies to manage stress effectively, engaging in regular physical activity, prioritizing quality sleep, adopting a balanced diet, practicing mindful eating, and seeking social support, we can support healthy cortisol regulation and promote weight management. Remember, individual factors, such as genetics and overall lifestyle, also contribute to weight management. Embrace a holistic approach, focusing on overall well-being, and consult with healthcare professionals for personalized guidance on your weight management journey.

Chapter 8: Can chronic stress lead to prolonged cortisol elevation?

We will explore the captivating connection between chronic stress and prolonged cortisol elevation. Cortisol, often referred to as the "stress hormone," is a vital component of our body's stress response. While cortisol is crucial for short-term survival, chronic or prolonged stress can lead to persistently elevated cortisol levels. In this chapter, we will delve into the fascinating realm of chronic stress and its impact on cortisol regulation, shedding light on the potential consequences and offering strategies for managing stress to promote a healthy cortisol balance.

Understanding Chronic Stress:

Before we delve into the relationship between chronic stress and cortisol, let's establish a clear understanding of what chronic stress entails. Chronic stress refers to a prolonged state of heightened psychological or emotional strain. It can be caused by various factors, such as work pressure, financial difficulties, relationship problems, or ongoing health issues. Unlike acute stress, which is short-lived and triggers immediate physiological responses, chronic stress persists over an extended period, leading to a continuous activation of the stress response system.

The HPA Axis and Cortisol Release:

To comprehend the relationship between chronic stress and cortisol elevation, we must first understand the hypothalamic-pituitary-adrenal (HPA) axis. The HPA axis is a complex network involving the hypothalamus, pituitary gland, and adrenal glands. It regulates the body's stress response and cortisol release.

During times of stress, the hypothalamus releases corticotropin-releasing hormone (CRH), which stimulates the pituitary gland to secrete adrenocorticotropic hormone (ACTH). ACTH then signals the adrenal glands to produce and release cortisol into the bloodstream. This cascade of events is a natural and adaptive response to acute stress, helping the body mobilize energy and resources to deal with the perceived threat.

Chronic Stress and Prolonged Cortisol Elevation:
While cortisol elevation is a necessary response to acute stress, chronic stress can disrupt the delicate balance of cortisol regulation. Prolonged exposure to stress can lead to persistently elevated cortisol levels, as the HPA axis remains activated for extended periods.

One mechanism underlying this prolonged cortisol elevation is dysregulation within the HPA axis. Chronic stress can disrupt the feedback loop that controls cortisol release, leading to excessive CRH and ACTH production and, consequently, increased cortisol secretion. This dysregulation can result from alterations in brain structure and function caused by chronic stress, impacting the hypothalamus and its ability to regulate cortisol release.

Consequences of Prolonged Cortisol Elevation:
Persistently elevated cortisol levels can have significant implications for our physical and mental well-being. Here are some consequences of prolonged cortisol elevation:

Impaired Immune Function:
Chronic stress and prolonged cortisol elevation can suppress immune system activity. While short-term cortisol increases immune readiness, long-term cortisol elevation weakens immune responses, making individuals more susceptible to infections and impairing wound healing.

Metabolic Imbalances:
Elevated cortisol levels can impact metabolism and contribute to weight gain, particularly abdominal fat accumulation. Chronic cortisol elevation can affect insulin sensitivity, leading to disrupted glucose metabolism and an increased risk of metabolic disorders such as type 2 diabetes.

Mood Disorders and Mental Health:
Persistently elevated cortisol levels have been associated with increased risk of mood disorders such as depression and anxiety. Chronic stress can disrupt the balance of neurotransmitters in the brain, affecting mood regulation and overall mental well-being.

Sleep Disruptions:
Chronic stress and high cortisol levels can interfere with sleep patterns. Sleep disturbances, such as difficulty falling asleep, staying

asleep, or poor sleep quality, are common in individuals experiencing chronic stress. Disrupted sleep can further exacerbate the effects of cortisol elevation, creating a cycle of stress and sleep disruptions.

Managing Chronic Stress and Cortisol Levels:

While it may not be possible to eliminate stress entirely from our lives, there are strategies to help manage chronic stress and promote a healthy cortisol balance:

Stress Management Techniques:

Incorporate stress management techniques into your daily routine. Engage in activities such as mindfulness meditation, deep breathing exercises, yoga, or engaging hobbies that promote relaxation and reduce stress. Regular practice can help regulate cortisol levels and enhance resilience in the face of stressors.

Social Support:

Maintain strong social connections and seek support from loved ones. Sharing your experiences and emotions with trusted individuals can help alleviate stress and buffer the impact of chronic stress on cortisol levels.

Healthy Lifestyle Habits:

Adopting a healthy lifestyle can support cortisol regulation and reduce the impact of chronic stress. Engage in regular physical activity, prioritize quality sleep, eat a balanced diet, and limit ... and caffeine intake. These habits provide a strong foundation for overall well-being and stress management.

Cognitive Behavioral Therapy (CBT):

CBT is a therapeutic approach that focuses on identifying and modifying unhelpful thoughts and behaviors. It can help individuals develop effective coping strategies for managing chronic stress, reduce the impact of stress on cortisol regulation, and improve overall mental well-being.

Time Management and Prioritization:

Organize your time effectively and prioritize tasks to minimize feelings of overwhelm and stress. Break larger tasks into smaller, manageable steps, delegate when possible, and set realistic goals. This approach can help reduce chronic stress and its impact on cortisol levels.

So,
Chronic stress can indeed lead to prolonged cortisol elevation, disrupting the delicate balance of cortisol regulation in the body. Persistently elevated cortisol levels have implications for immune function, metabolism, mental health, and sleep patterns. By implementing strategies for managing chronic stress, such as stress management techniques, social support, healthy lifestyle habits, and seeking professional help if needed, we can promote a healthy cortisol balance and enhance overall well-being. Remember, managing chronic stress is a journey that requires patience, self-compassion, and a commitment to self-care.

Chapter 9: How does cortisol affect memory and cognitive function?

We will explore the intriguing connection between cortisol and memory and cognitive function. Cortisol, known as the "stress hormone," plays a crucial role in our body's response to stress. However, its influence extends beyond the stress response and into our cognitive abilities. In this chapter, we will delve into the fascinating ways in which cortisol impacts memory and cognitive function, shedding light on its effects and offering strategies to support cognitive well-being.

Understanding Memory and Cognitive Function:

Before we dive into the specifics of cortisol's impact, let's establish a foundation of memory and cognitive function. Memory encompasses the processes involved in encoding, storing, and retrieving information. Cognitive function refers to the mental abilities associated with attention, perception, learning, problem-solving, and decision-making. These cognitive processes are essential for our daily functioning and overall well-being.

Cortisol and Memory Formation:

Cortisol can influence memory formation, particularly in relation to stressful experiences. Acute stress triggers the release of cortisol, which, in moderation, can enhance memory consolidation of emotionally significant events. This mechanism helps us remember potentially threatening or important information in the future, aiding in our survival and adaptation.

However, prolonged, or chronic cortisol elevation can have detrimental effects on memory. High levels of cortisol can impair memory retrieval and the consolidation of non-emotional information. This can lead to difficulties in remembering details, reduced attention span, and decreased overall cognitive performance.

Cortisol and Hippocampal Function:

The hippocampus, a brain structure vital for memory formation and consolidation, is highly sensitive to cortisol. Prolonged exposure to high levels of cortisol can have negative implications for hippocampal function. Here's how cortisol affects the hippocampus:

Hippocampal Volume: Chronic cortisol elevation has been associated with reduced hippocampal volume, which can impact memory and cognitive abilities. The hippocampus plays a crucial role in transferring information from short-term to long-term memory, and its structural integrity is vital for optimal memory function.

Neuroplasticity: Cortisol can affect the neuroplasticity of the hippocampus, influencing the formation of new connections between brain cells. Impaired neuroplasticity due to prolonged cortisol elevation can hinder the brain's ability to adapt, learn, and form new memories.

Neural Communication: Cortisol can alter the communication between brain cells in the hippocampus. It can affect the balance of neurotransmitters involved in memory and cognitive function, such as glutamate and gamma-aminobutyric acid (GABA). Disrupted neural communication can impair memory encoding and retrieval processes.

Cortisol and Cognitive Function:

In addition to its impact on memory, cortisol can also affect other aspects of cognitive function. Here are some key areas influenced by cortisol:

Attention and Focus: Prolonged cortisol elevation can interfere with attention and concentration. Individuals experiencing chronic stress may have difficulties staying focused and may find their attention easily shifting from task to task.

Decision-Making: Cortisol can influence decision-making processes. High cortisol levels have been associated with a tendency to make more conservative or risk-averse decisions, potentially impacting problem-solving abilities and adaptability.

Working Memory: Working memory, the cognitive system responsible for temporarily holding and manipulating information, can be affected by cortisol. Elevated cortisol levels can impair working memory capacity, making it challenging to hold and process information in the mind.

Strategies to Support Memory and Cognitive Function:

While cortisol's impact on memory and cognitive function can be challenging, there are strategies to support cognitive well-being:

Stress Management:

Effectively managing stress can help regulate cortisol levels and minimize its impact on memory and cognitive function. Engage in stress-reducing activities such as mindfulness meditation, deep breathing exercises, and engaging hobbies that promote relaxation and reduce stress.

Regular Physical Activity:

Exercise has numerous benefits for brain health and cognitive function. Engaging in regular physical activity, such as aerobic exercises or strength training, promotes blood flow to the brain and supports the growth and connectivity of brain cells.

Mental Stimulation:

Keep your mind active and engaged. Engage in activities that challenge your cognitive abilities, such as puzzles, reading, learning a new skill, or playing musical instruments. Mental stimulation promotes neuroplasticity and can help counteract the negative effects of cortisol on memory and cognitive function.

Healthy Lifestyle Habits:

Adopting a healthy lifestyle that includes a balanced diet, adequate sleep, and social engagement can support cognitive function. A nutritious diet rich in antioxidants, omega-3 fatty acids, and vitamins supports brain health. Quality sleep and social interactions also contribute to cognitive well-being.

Memory Techniques:

Explore memory-enhancing techniques such as visualization, association, and repetition. These techniques can help improve memory encoding and retrieval processes. Consider using memory aids, such as calendars, reminders, or note-taking apps, to support information organization and retention.

Cognitive Training:

Participate in cognitive training programs designed to improve memory and cognitive function. These programs typically involve engaging in structured exercises and tasks that challenge different cognitive abilities, helping to enhance overall cognitive performance.

So,

Cortisol plays a significant role in memory and cognitive function. While acute cortisol release can enhance memory consolidation of emotionally significant events, chronic or prolonged cortisol elevation can have negative effects on memory, attention, decision-making, and overall cognitive performance.

By managing stress effectively, engaging in regular physical activity, seeking mental stimulation, adopting healthy lifestyle habits, and utilizing memory-enhancing techniques, we can support memory and cognitive function. Remember, every individual is unique, and finding the strategies that work best for you is essential. Embrace a holistic approach to brain health and be patient with yourself as you explore different techniques and strategies. With a proactive approach to managing cortisol and supporting cognitive well-being, you can optimize your memory and cognitive function for a fulfilling and enriching life.

Chapter 10: What are the long-term effects of high cortisol levels on overall health?

We will explore the long-term effects of high cortisol levels on overall health. Cortisol, known as the "stress hormone," plays a crucial role in our body's response to stress. While cortisol is necessary for our survival in the short term, chronically elevated levels can have detrimental effects on our well-being. In this chapter, we will delve into the fascinating realm of high cortisol levels and their impact on various aspects of overall health, shedding light on the potential consequences and offering strategies for managing cortisol to promote long-term wellness.

Understanding Cortisol and Its Functions:

Before we dive into the details, let's establish a basic understanding of cortisol and its functions in the body. Cortisol is a hormone produced by the adrenal glands, which sit atop the kidneys. It is involved in numerous physiological processes, including:

Stress Response: Cortisol helps our body respond to stress by mobilizing energy, increasing blood sugar levels, and enhancing alertness.

Metabolism: Cortisol influences metabolism by regulating glucose levels, promoting the breakdown of stored glycogen, and facilitating the release of fatty acids for energy.

Inflammation Regulation: Cortisol has anti-inflammatory properties, helping to suppress excessive inflammation in the body.

Immune Function: Cortisol plays a role in modulating immune responses, regulating the intensity and duration of immune reactions.

Long-Term Effects of High Cortisol Levels:

While cortisol is essential for our body's functioning, prolonged elevation of cortisol levels can have detrimental effects on overall health. Here are some long-term consequences of high cortisol levels:

Impaired Immune Function:

Chronically elevated cortisol levels can suppress immune system function. This can lead to an increased susceptibility to infections, slower wound healing, and a higher risk of developing autoimmune disorders.

Increased Risk of Cardiovascular Disease:

High cortisol levels have been associated with an increased risk of cardiovascular disease. Prolonged cortisol elevation can contribute to elevated blood pressure, impaired lipid metabolism, insulin resistance, and abdominal obesity—all of which are risk factors for heart disease.

Impaired Cognitive Function:

Persistently elevated cortisol levels can have negative effects on cognitive function. High cortisol has been linked to impaired memory, reduced attention span, difficulty concentrating, and cognitive decline over time.

Metabolic Imbalances:

Chronic elevation of cortisol can disrupt metabolic processes, leading to imbalances that contribute to weight gain, particularly in the abdominal region. High cortisol levels can affect insulin sensitivity, promoting glucose intolerance and increasing the risk of developing type 2 diabetes.

Bone Density Loss:

Long-term exposure to high cortisol levels can contribute to bone density loss and increase the risk of osteoporosis. Cortisol can interfere with bone formation and remodeling, leading to weakened bones and an increased susceptibility to fractures.

Mood Disorders and Mental Health:

Persistently elevated cortisol levels have been associated with an increased risk of mood disorders such as depression and anxiety. Chronic stress and high cortisol can disrupt neurotransmitter balance, impacting mood regulation and overall mental well-being.

Managing Cortisol and Promoting Long-Term Wellness:

While high cortisol levels can have adverse effects on overall health, there are strategies to manage cortisol and promote long-term wellness:

Stress Management:

Effective stress management techniques play a crucial role in regulating cortisol levels. Engage in activities such as mindfulness meditation, deep breathing exercises, yoga, or engaging hobbies that promote relaxation and reduce stress. Regular practice can help modulate cortisol and enhance resilience in the face of stressors.

Regular Physical Activity:

Exercise has numerous benefits for overall health, including cortisol regulation. Engaging in regular physical activity, such as aerobic exercises or strength training, helps reduce cortisol levels, promote metabolic balance, and enhance well-being.

Healthy Lifestyle Habits:

Adopting a healthy lifestyle supports cortisol regulation and overall well-being. Focus on a balanced diet rich in fruits, vegetables, whole grains, and lean proteins. Prioritize quality sleep, limit ... and caffeine intake, and foster social connections to reduce stress and promote hormonal balance.

Mindfulness and Relaxation Techniques:

Incorporate mindfulness and relaxation techniques into your daily routine. Practices such as meditation, deep breathing exercises, progressive muscle relaxation, or spending time in nature can help lower cortisol levels and promote a sense of calm.

Social Support:

Maintaining strong social connections and seeking support from loved ones is crucial for managing stress and cortisol levels. Share your experiences and emotions with trusted individuals who can provide encouragement, understanding, and help alleviate stress.

Seek Professional Help:

If you're struggling with chronic stress or high cortisol levels, consider seeking professional help. Healthcare providers, such as doctors, therapists, or endocrinologists, can provide guidance, support, and tailored interventions to help manage cortisol and promote long-term wellness.

So,

High cortisol levels, if left unmanaged, can have significant long-term effects on overall health. Impaired immune function, increased risk of cardiovascular disease, cognitive decline, metabolic imbalances, bone density loss, and mood disorders are among the potential consequences of chronic cortisol elevation.

By adopting strategies to manage stress effectively, engaging in regular physical activity, prioritizing healthy lifestyle habits, practicing mindfulness and relaxation techniques, fostering social support, and seeking professional help when needed, we can support cortisol regulation and promote long-term wellness. Remember, each person is unique, and finding the right combination of strategies that work for you is important. Embrace a holistic approach to your health, prioritize self-care, and take proactive steps to manage cortisol for a balanced and thriving life.

Chapter 11: Is there a connection between cortisol and anxiety disorders?

We will explore the intriguing connection between cortisol and anxiety disorders. Anxiety disorders are among the most common mental health conditions, affecting millions of people worldwide. Cortisol, the "stress hormone," plays a vital role in our body's stress response. In this chapter, we will delve into the fascinating realm of cortisol and anxiety, shedding light on the potential connection between the two and offering insights into the complex interplay between cortisol and anxiety disorders.

Understanding Anxiety Disorders:

Before we delve into the specifics of the cortisol-anxiety relationship, let's establish a foundational understanding of anxiety disorders. Anxiety disorders are a group of mental health conditions characterized by excessive and persistent worry, fear, or apprehension. Common types of anxiety disorders include generalized anxiety disorder (GAD), panic disorder, social anxiety disorder, and specific phobias.

Cortisol and the Stress Response:

Cortisol plays a key role in our body's response to stress. When faced with a perceived threat, the brain triggers the release of cortisol, preparing the body for a fight-or-flight response. Cortisol mobilizes energy, increases blood sugar levels, and enhances alertness, helping us respond to the stressor effectively.

The Cortisol-Anxiety Connection:

While cortisol is crucial for our survival in the face of acute stress, its chronic dysregulation can contribute to anxiety disorders. Here are some ways in which cortisol and anxiety are connected:

Dysregulated Stress Response:

In individuals with anxiety disorders, the stress response system may be dysregulated, leading to excessive cortisol release even in non-threatening situations. This dysregulation can result from factors such as genetics, past traumatic experiences, or heightened sensitivity to stress. Elevated cortisol levels can exacerbate anxiety symptoms and contribute to a heightened state of arousal.

Altered Cortisol Patterns:

Research has shown that individuals with anxiety disorders may exhibit altered cortisol patterns compared to those without anxiety. For example, some studies have observed higher baseline cortisol levels in individuals with GAD. Others have reported abnormal cortisol awakening responses, where cortisol levels fail to rise as expected upon waking, in individuals with various anxiety disorders.

Interaction with Neurotransmitters:

Cortisol interacts with various neurotransmitters in the brain, including serotonin and gamma-aminobutyric acid (GABA), which are involved in mood regulation. Dysregulated cortisol levels can impact the balance of these neurotransmitters, potentially contributing to anxiety symptoms.

Feedback Loop Disruption:

Cortisol is regulated by a feedback loop involving the hypothalamus, pituitary gland, and adrenal glands. In individuals with anxiety disorders, this feedback loop may be disrupted, leading to higher cortisol levels. The dysregulation of this feedback loop can contribute to a chronic state of anxiety and physiological hyperarousal.

Impact on Hippocampus:

The hippocampus, a brain region involved in emotion regulation and memory formation, is highly sensitive to cortisol. Elevated cortisol levels can have adverse effects on the hippocampus, potentially impairing its functioning. This can contribute to difficulties in emotional regulation and the formation of fear-based memories, which are often characteristic of anxiety disorders.

Managing Cortisol and Anxiety:

While the connection between cortisol and anxiety is complex, there are strategies to help manage cortisol levels and alleviate anxiety symptoms:

Stress Management Techniques:

Effective stress management techniques play a crucial role in regulating cortisol and reducing anxiety. Engage in activities such as mindfulness meditation, deep breathing exercises, yoga, or engaging hobbies that promote relaxation and reduce stress. Regular practice can help modulate cortisol levels and enhance resilience in the face of anxiety-provoking situations.

Cognitive Behavioral Therapy (CBT):

CBT is a widely recognized therapeutic approach for anxiety disorders. It focuses on identifying and modifying unhelpful thought patterns and behaviors. CBT can help individuals challenge anxious thoughts, develop coping strategies, and gradually confront feared situations, reducing anxiety symptoms and improving overall well-being.

Medication:

In some cases, healthcare professionals may prescribe medications, such as selective serotonin reuptake inhibitors (SSRIs) or benzodiazepines, to manage anxiety symptoms. These medications can help regulate neurotransmitter levels, including serotonin and GABA, and may indirectly impact cortisol regulation.

Healthy Lifestyle Habits:

Adopting a healthy lifestyle can support cortisol regulation and overall well-being. Prioritize regular physical activity, eat a balanced diet rich in fruits, vegetables, whole grains, and lean proteins, get adequate sleep, limit ... and caffeine intake, and foster social connections. These habits contribute to stress reduction and promote hormonal balance.

Social Support:

Maintaining strong social connections and seeking support from loved ones can help alleviate anxiety symptoms and buffer the impact of stress on cortisol levels. Share your experiences and emotions with trusted individuals who can provide understanding, encouragement, and assistance in navigating anxiety challenges.

Mindfulness and Relaxation Techniques:

Incorporate mindfulness and relaxation techniques into your daily routine. Practices such as meditation, deep breathing exercises, progressive muscle relaxation, or engaging in hobbies that promote relaxation can help lower cortisol levels and promote a sense of calm. So,

While the connection between cortisol and anxiety disorders is complex, evidence suggests a potential relationship between the two. Dysregulated cortisol levels, altered stress response, disrupted feedback loop, and interaction with neurotransmitters are among the factors contributing to the cortisol-anxiety connection.

By implementing strategies for stress management, engaging in therapy, adopting healthy lifestyle habits, seeking social support, and practicing mindfulness and relaxation techniques, individuals with anxiety disorders can support cortisol regulation and alleviate anxiety symptoms. Remember, managing anxiety is a unique journey, and it may involve a combination of approaches tailored to your specific needs. Be patient with yourself, seek professional guidance when needed, and prioritize self-care to promote a balanced and fulfilling life, free from the constraints of anxiety.

Chapter 12: Can cortisol levels be measured accurately through saliva or blood tests?

We will explore the fascinating topic of measuring cortisol levels through saliva and blood tests. Cortisol, known as the "stress hormone," plays a crucial role in our body's stress response and various physiological processes. Measuring cortisol levels can provide valuable insights into hormonal balance, stress levels, and overall health. In this chapter, we will delve into the details of cortisol testing, discussing the accuracy and benefits of saliva and blood tests, and how they can be used to assess cortisol levels.

Understanding Cortisol Testing:

Cortisol testing involves the measurement of cortisol levels in biological samples such as saliva or blood. These tests provide an objective assessment of cortisol levels, offering valuable information about the body's stress response and hormonal balance. Let's explore two common methods of cortisol testing: saliva and blood tests.

Saliva Tests:

Saliva testing, also known as salivary cortisol testing, measures cortisol levels in the saliva. It offers several advantages and is increasingly utilized in clinical and research settings. Here's what you need to know about saliva tests:

Non-Invasive and Convenient:

Saliva testing is non-invasive and can be performed in the comfort of your own home or a healthcare professional's office. It involves collecting a saliva sample using a swab or small collection tube.

Diurnal Cortisol Pattern Assessment:

Saliva testing allows for the assessment of diurnal cortisol patterns, which refer to the natural fluctuation of cortisol levels throughout the day. Multiple samples are collected at specific times (typically morning, afternoon, and evening) to assess the cortisol awakening response and diurnal rhythm.

Ease of Collection and Storage:

Saliva collection is relatively simple and can be performed by individuals themselves. The samples are stable and can be stored at room temperature for a certain period, making them convenient for transport and analysis.

Lower Cost:

Compared to blood tests, saliva testing is generally less expensive, making it a more accessible option for cortisol assessment.

Blood Tests:

Blood tests are another method used to measure cortisol levels. They involve the collection of a blood sample, typically from a vein in the arm. Here are some important aspects of blood tests for cortisol measurement:

Direct Measurement of Total Cortisol:

Blood tests directly measure the total cortisol levels in the bloodstream. They provide an accurate assessment of cortisol levels at a specific point in time.

Laboratory-Based Analysis:

Blood samples need to be processed in a laboratory using specialized equipment. This may require a visit to a healthcare facility or a laboratory for sample collection and analysis.

Clinically Established Reference Ranges:

Blood cortisol levels are often compared to established reference ranges to determine if they fall within the normal range or if further investigation is necessary. These reference ranges are based on population averages and provide a benchmark for assessment.

Acute Stress Response Assessment:

Blood tests are particularly useful in situations where immediate cortisol measurement is necessary, such as in emergencies or when assessing acute stress responses.

Accuracy of Saliva and Blood Tests:

Both saliva and blood tests can provide accurate measurements of cortisol levels when performed correctly. However, it's important to note that various factors can influence cortisol levels, leading to variations in test results. Here are some considerations:

Diurnal Variation:

Cortisol levels naturally fluctuate throughout the day, with the highest levels typically in the morning upon waking and gradually decreasing as the day progresses. The diurnal rhythm should be considered when interpreting test results.

Sampling Technique:

Proper technique is crucial for accurate results. Follow the instructions provided with the testing kit or consult a healthcare professional to ensure correct saliva or blood sample collection.

Interference Factors:

Certain medications, substances (such as caffeine or nicotine), and medical conditions can potentially affect cortisol levels and may need to be considered when interpreting test results.

Laboratory Standards and Calibration:

Ensure that the laboratory conducting the analysis follows established quality control standards and calibration procedures to ensure accurate and reliable results.

Choosing the Right Test for Your Needs:

The choice between saliva and blood testing depends on various factors, including the purpose of testing, convenience, and the information you seek. Saliva testing is often preferred for assessing diurnal cortisol patterns and monitoring chronic stress levels, while blood testing is commonly used for immediate cortisol assessment and in clinical settings.

It's important to consult with a healthcare professional to determine the most suitable testing method for your specific situation and to interpret the results accurately in the context of your overall health and well-being.

So,

Measuring cortisol levels through saliva and blood tests offers valuable insights into hormonal balance, stress levels, and overall health. Saliva testing provides a non-invasive and convenient option for assessing diurnal cortisol patterns and chronic stress levels. On the other hand, blood testing directly measures total cortisol levels and is useful for immediate assessment and in clinical settings.

Both saliva and blood tests can provide accurate measurements when performed correctly, considering factors such as diurnal variation, sampling technique, interference factors, and laboratory standards. To choose the right test for your needs, consult with a healthcare professional who can guide you based on your specific circumstances. Remember, cortisol testing is just one piece of the puzzle in assessing overall health and stress levels. It's important to consider test results in the context of your symptoms, medical history, and lifestyle factors. By utilizing cortisol testing appropriately, you can gain valuable insights and work towards optimizing your well-being and managing stress effectively.

Chapter 13: How does cortisol impact the reproductive system in men and women?

We will explore the fascinating impact of cortisol, the "stress hormone," on the reproductive system in both men and women. While cortisol is primarily known for its role in the stress response, it also influences various physiological processes, including reproduction. In this chapter, we will delve into the details of how cortisol affects the reproductive system, shedding light on its effects on fertility, hormone balance, and sexual health.

Understanding the Reproductive System:

Before we dive into the specifics of cortisol's impact, let's establish a foundational understanding of the reproductive system in men and women. The reproductive system encompasses organs, hormones, and processes that enable conception, pregnancy, and childbirth. In women, key components include the ovaries, fallopian tubes, uterus, and vagina, while men have testes, seminal vesicles, prostate gland, and penis.

Cortisol and Female Reproductive System:

Cortisol can exert notable effects on the female reproductive system. Here are some key areas of impact:

Menstrual Cycle Irregularities:

High levels of cortisol can disrupt the delicate hormonal balance necessary for regular menstrual cycles. Chronic stress and elevated cortisol levels may lead to menstrual irregularities, such as irregular or absent periods, shorter or longer cycles, and anovulation (lack of ovulation).

Fertility:

Cortisol can impact fertility by interfering with the reproductive hormone cascade. Elevated cortisol levels can disrupt the balance of hormones involved in ovulation and fertility, potentially leading to difficulties in conceiving.

Polycystic Ovary Syndrome (PCOS):

Chronic stress and high cortisol levels may contribute to the development or exacerbation of polycystic ovary syndrome (PCOS).

PCOS is a hormonal disorder characterized by irregular periods, cysts on the ovaries, and excess androgen (male hormone) production. Cortisol dysregulation can disrupt hormone production, exacerbating PCOS symptoms.

Sexual Desire and Arousal:

Elevated cortisol levels can affect sexual desire and arousal in women. Chronic stress and cortisol dysregulation may lead to reduced libido and difficulties with sexual responsiveness.

Cortisol and Male Reproductive System:

Cortisol also impacts the male reproductive system. Here are some key areas of impact:

Testosterone Production:

Cortisol and testosterone have an inverse relationship. When cortisol levels are elevated, testosterone levels tend to decrease. Chronic stress and high cortisol levels can interfere with testosterone production, potentially leading to reduced libido, erectile dysfunction, and impaired sperm production.

Sperm Quality and Fertility:

Elevated cortisol levels can negatively affect sperm quality and fertility in men. Studies have shown that chronic stress and cortisol dysregulation can lead to reduced sperm motility, lower sperm count, and abnormal sperm morphology, making it more difficult to achieve conception.

Erectile Dysfunction:

Cortisol dysregulation can contribute to erectile dysfunction (ED) in men. Chronic stress and high cortisol levels may impair blood flow to the penis and affect the ability to achieve and maintain an erection.

Managing Cortisol and Promoting Reproductive Health:

While cortisol's impact on the reproductive system can be challenging, there are strategies to manage cortisol levels and promote reproductive health in both men and women:

Stress Management Techniques:

Effective stress management techniques play a crucial role in regulating cortisol levels and promoting reproductive health. Engage in activities such as mindfulness meditation, deep breathing exercises, yoga, or engaging hobbies that promote relaxation and reduce stress. Regular practice can help modulate cortisol levels and enhance overall well-being.

Healthy Lifestyle Habits:

Adopting a healthy lifestyle can support cortisol regulation and reproductive health. Focus on a balanced diet rich in fruits, vegetables, whole grains, and lean proteins. Prioritize regular physical activity, adequate sleep, limit ... and caffeine intake, and foster social connections. These habits contribute to stress reduction and promote hormonal balance.

Communication and Intimacy:

Maintaining open communication and emotional intimacy with your partner can help reduce stress levels and promote a supportive environment for reproductive health. Discussing concerns and seeking emotional support can alleviate stress and improve overall well-being.

Seeking Professional Help:

If you're experiencing difficulties with fertility, sexual health, or suspect cortisol dysregulation, it's essential to seek professional help. Healthcare professionals, such as gynecologists, urologists, or reproductive endocrinologists, can provide guidance, perform necessary evaluations, and recommend appropriate treatments or interventions tailored to your specific needs.

Fertility and Sexual Health Support:

For individuals struggling with fertility or sexual health issues, there are various medical interventions available, including assisted reproductive technologies, hormone therapy, and counseling. Seeking guidance from fertility specialists, sexual health experts, or therapists can provide additional support and guidance on the best course of action.

So,

Cortisol, the stress hormone, can significantly impact the reproductive system in both men and women. Elevated cortisol levels and chronic stress can disrupt hormonal balance, leading to menstrual irregularities, fertility issues, reduced libido, erectile dysfunction, and impaired sperm quality. However, by implementing strategies for managing cortisol, adopting a healthy lifestyle, prioritizing stress management techniques, fostering open communication, and seeking professional help when needed, individuals can support cortisol regulation and promote reproductive health.

Remember, each person's reproductive health journey is unique, and it may involve a combination of approaches tailored to their specific needs. Be patient with yourself, seek appropriate support, and prioritize self-care to optimize your reproductive well-being. By managing cortisol levels and promoting a balanced lifestyle, you can enhance your chances of maintaining reproductive health and overall well-being.

Chapter 14: What is the cortisol awakening response and its significance?

We will explore the intriguing concept of the cortisol awakening response (CAR) and its significance. Cortisol, the "stress hormone," plays a crucial role in our body's stress response and various physiological processes. The cortisol awakening response refers to the natural increase in cortisol levels upon awakening in the morning. In this chapter, we will delve into the details of CAR, shedding light on its physiological mechanisms, its significance in regulating our daily rhythm, and its potential implications for health and well-being.

Understanding the Cortisol Awakening Response:

The cortisol awakening response is a distinct pattern of cortisol release that occurs in the early morning hours upon awakening. Let's explore the key aspects of CAR:

Timing of the Response:

The cortisol awakening response typically occurs within the first 30 to 45 minutes after waking up. It represents a rapid increase in cortisol levels that can be observed in saliva or blood samples collected during this period.

Magnitude of the Response:

The cortisol awakening response involves a significant increase in cortisol levels compared to the levels present prior to awakening. Studies have shown that the magnitude of the CAR can be two to three times higher than the average cortisol level during the rest of the day.

Individual Variation:

The magnitude of the cortisol awakening response can vary among individuals. Some people exhibit a robust response, while others may have a more muted or blunted response. Factors such as age, sex, genetics, and lifestyle factors can contribute to the variability observed.

Physiological Mechanisms of the Cortisol Awakening Response:

The cortisol awakening response is regulated by a complex interplay between the hypothalamus, pituitary gland, and adrenal glands. Here's a breakdown of the physiological mechanisms involved:

Hypothalamic-Pituitary-Adrenal (HPA) Axis Activation:

Upon awakening, the brain's hypothalamus releases corticotropin-releasing hormone (CRH), which stimulates the pituitary gland to release adrenocorticotropic hormone (ACTH). ACTH, in turn, signals the adrenal glands to release cortisol into the bloodstream.

Sensitivity to Anticipation and External Cues:

The cortisol awakening response is influenced by anticipation and external cues associated with waking up. Factors such as the anticipation of the day's tasks, social interactions, and the start of daily routines can trigger the activation of the HPA axis and subsequent cortisol release.

Neural and Endocrine Regulation:

Multiple neural and endocrine factors influence the cortisol awakening response. The suprachiasmatic nucleus (SCN), a master circadian clock located in the brain's hypothalamus, plays a role in regulating the timing of the response. Additionally, interactions between cortisol and neurotransmitters, such as dopamine and norepinephrine, may modulate the magnitude of the response.

Significance of the Cortisol Awakening Response:

The cortisol awakening response serves several important functions and has significant implications for our daily rhythm, health, and well-being. Let's explore its significance:

Regulation of the Circadian Rhythm:

The cortisol awakening response helps synchronize our internal body clock, known as the circadian rhythm. It provides an essential signal to the body that it's time to transition from rest to activity, preparing us for the demands of the day.

Energy Mobilization and Alertness:

The rapid increase in cortisol levels upon awakening is thought to mobilize energy stores, increase blood sugar levels, and enhance alertness. This surge in cortisol supports the body's readiness to engage in daily activities and meet the challenges of the day.

Psychosocial Adaptation and Coping:

The cortisol awakening response is influenced by psychosocial factors, including stress, mood, and anticipation. Research suggests that the magnitude of the response may reflect an individual's psychosocial adaptation and coping abilities, providing insight into their resilience and response to daily stressors.

Diurnal Cortisol Patterns:

The cortisol awakening response contributes to the diurnal cortisol pattern, which refers to the natural fluctuation of cortisol levels throughout the day. The response represents the initial surge in cortisol levels, followed by a gradual decline as the day progresses. The diurnal cortisol pattern helps maintain the body's balance and prepares it for restorative sleep at night.

Clinical and Research Implications:

The cortisol awakening response has garnered attention in clinical and research settings due to its potential implications for health and well-being. Here are some areas where the CAR is of interest:

Stress Research:

The cortisol awakening response is sensitive to psychosocial stressors, making it a valuable tool for studying the impact of stress on the body. Researchers can assess how stressors influence the magnitude and timing of the response, providing insights into individual stress reactivity and adaptation.

Mood Disorders and Psychological Health:

Alterations in the cortisol awakening response have been observed in individuals with mood disorders such as depression and anxiety. Blunted or exaggerated responses may reflect dysregulation of the HPA axis and potential vulnerability to these conditions.

Chronobiology and Sleep Disorders:

The cortisol awakening response is intricately connected to the body's circadian rhythm and the sleep-wake cycle. Abnormal CAR patterns have been associated with sleep disorders such as insomnia and shift work-related sleep disturbances. Evaluating the cortisol awakening response can aid in understanding these conditions and developing targeted interventions.

Psychophysiological Research:

The cortisol awakening response is a useful tool for investigating the interplay between the mind and body. Researchers can examine how psychological factors, such as cognitive processes, emotion regulation, and social context, influence the CAR and vice versa.

So,

The cortisol awakening response represents the rapid increase in cortisol levels upon awakening, playing a significant role in regulating our daily rhythm, energy mobilization, and psychosocial adaptation. It is a complex physiological response influenced by anticipation, external cues, and the interplay of neural and endocrine factors.

Understanding the significance of the cortisol awakening response provides insights into our circadian rhythm, stress response, and potential implications for health and well-being. Researchers and clinicians utilize the CAR to explore stress reactivity, mood disorders, sleep disturbances, and psychophysiological processes.

By unraveling the intricacies of the cortisol awakening response, we deepen our understanding of the body's stress response system and its impact on our daily lives. Embracing this knowledge allows us to appreciate the interconnections between our internal rhythms, stress resilience, and overall well-being.

Chapter 15: Can cortisol levels be regulated through mindfulness practices?

We will explore the intriguing relationship between mindfulness practices and cortisol regulation. Cortisol, known as the "stress hormone," plays a crucial role in our body's stress response. Mindfulness practices, such as meditation and mindful awareness, have gained popularity for their potential to reduce stress and enhance well-being. In this chapter, we will delve into the details of how mindfulness practices can influence cortisol levels, shedding light on the mechanisms involved and offering insights into incorporating mindfulness into daily life for stress reduction and cortisol regulation.

Understanding Cortisol and Stress Response:

Before we dive into the specifics of mindfulness and cortisol regulation, let's establish a foundational understanding of cortisol and the stress response. Cortisol is a hormone produced by the adrenal glands in response to stress. It mobilizes energy, increases blood sugar levels, and enhances alertness, preparing our body for the challenges we face.

The stress response is crucial for our survival in acute situations, but chronic stress and elevated cortisol levels can have adverse effects on our physical and mental well-being. Chronic stress has been linked to various health issues, including cardiovascular problems, impaired immune function, mood disorders, and cognitive difficulties.

Mindfulness and Cortisol Regulation:

Mindfulness practices involve bringing attention to the present moment, cultivating non-judgmental awareness, and developing an attitude of acceptance and compassion. Research suggests that these practices can influence cortisol levels and contribute to cortisol regulation. Here's how mindfulness practices can impact cortisol:

Stress Reduction:

Mindfulness practices are effective in reducing stress levels. By focusing attention on the present moment and cultivating an attitude of acceptance, mindfulness helps individuals disengage from ruminative thoughts and worries about the past or future. This shift in focus can alleviate psychological distress, thereby reducing the release of stress hormones, including cortisol.

Modulating the Stress Response:

Mindfulness practices have been found to modulate the physiological stress response. By training individuals to observe their bodily sensations, thoughts, and emotions without judgment, mindfulness can enhance self-regulation and promote adaptive coping strategies. This can lead to a decreased activation of the stress response system, resulting in lower cortisol levels.

Mindful Coping with Stressors:

Practicing mindfulness allows individuals to approach stressors with greater equanimity and resilience. By developing an accepting and non-reactive stance, individuals can respond to stressors in a more measured and calm manner, reducing the likelihood of an excessive cortisol response.

Enhancing Emotional Regulation:

Mindfulness practices promote emotional regulation by increasing awareness of emotions and cultivating a non-judgmental attitude toward them. This enhanced emotional regulation can prevent prolonged activation of the stress response and help maintain cortisol levels within a healthy range.

Improving Sleep Quality:

Mindfulness practices have been shown to improve sleep quality, which, in turn, can impact cortisol levels. Restful sleep supports the body's natural cortisol regulation, ensuring a healthy cortisol awakening response and maintaining the diurnal cortisol rhythm.

Incorporating Mindfulness into Daily Life:

To harness the benefits of mindfulness for cortisol regulation, consider incorporating the following practices into your daily life:

Formal Meditation:

Set aside dedicated time each day for formal meditation practice. Find a quiet space, sit comfortably, and focus your attention on your breath, bodily sensations, or a chosen meditation object. Start with a few minutes and gradually increase the duration as you become more comfortable.

Mindful Awareness:

Bring mindfulness into everyday activities by engaging in them with full presence and attention. Whether you're eating, walking, or engaging in routine tasks, bring awareness to the sensations, thoughts, and emotions that arise in the present moment.

Body Scan:

Practice a body scan meditation, where you systematically bring attention to different parts of your body, observing sensations without judgment. This practice promotes a deep sense of relaxation and body awareness, reducing cortisol levels and promoting overall well-being.

Mindful Breathing:

Engage in mindful breathing exercises throughout the day. Take a few moments to focus on your breath, observing the inhalation and exhalation without trying to change anything. This simple practice can help regulate stress and cortisol levels in the midst of daily challenges.

Mindful Movement:

Incorporate mindful movement practices such as yoga, tai chi, or qigong into your routine. These practices combine gentle physical movements with focused attention, promoting relaxation, stress reduction, and cortisol regulation.

Mindful Self-Compassion:

Develop self-compassion by treating yourself with kindness and understanding. When faced with stress or self-criticism, offer yourself words of compassion and practice self-care. Self-compassion practices can help buffer the impact of stress on cortisol levels and enhance overall well-being.

So,

Mindfulness practices have shown promise in influencing cortisol levels and promoting cortisol regulation. By reducing stress, modulating the stress response, enhancing emotional regulation, and improving sleep quality, mindfulness can contribute to a healthier cortisol profile.

Incorporating mindfulness into daily life through formal meditation, mindful awareness, body scan, mindful breathing, mindful movement, and self-compassion practices empowers individuals to cultivate present-moment awareness, reduce stress, and enhance well-being. With regular practice and patience, mindfulness can become a valuable tool for stress reduction and cortisol regulation, supporting overall physical and mental health.

Remember, each person's mindfulness journey is unique, and finding the practices that resonate with you is important. Embrace a gentle and non-judgmental approach as you explore mindfulness and allow the benefits to unfold gradually. By cultivating mindfulness and regulating cortisol, you can navigate life's challenges with greater equanimity and promote a sense of inner calm and balance.

Chapter 16: How does cortisol affect bone health and osteoporosis risk?

We will explore the fascinating connection between cortisol and bone health, specifically its impact on osteoporosis risk. Osteoporosis is a condition characterized by weakened and brittle bones, making them more susceptible to fractures. Cortisol, the "stress hormone," plays a crucial role in our body's stress response and various physiological processes. In this chapter, we will delve into the details of how cortisol affects bone health, shedding light on the mechanisms involved and offering insights into managing cortisol to promote optimal bone health and reduce osteoporosis risk.

Understanding Cortisol and its Role in the Body:

Before we dive into the specifics of cortisol and bone health, let's establish a foundational understanding of cortisol and its role in the body. Cortisol is a hormone produced by the adrenal glands in response to stress. It is involved in numerous physiological processes, including metabolism, immune function, and the body's stress response.

Cortisol and Bone Remodeling:

Bone remodeling is a dynamic process that involves the constant breakdown and formation of bone tissue. It helps maintain bone strength and adapt to mechanical stress. Cortisol can influence bone remodeling by affecting the activity of bone cells, including osteoblasts (responsible for bone formation) and osteoclasts (responsible for bone resorption). Here's how cortisol impacts bone health:

Increased Bone Resorption:

Elevated cortisol levels can stimulate bone resorption, leading to increased breakdown of bone tissue. Cortisol promotes the differentiation and activity of osteoclasts, resulting in higher bone resorption rates. Prolonged or excessive cortisol exposure can disrupt the balance between bone formation and resorption, leading to a net loss of bone mass.

Decreased Bone Formation:

Cortisol can inhibit the activity of osteoblasts, reducing their ability to form new bone tissue. This can result in reduced bone mineral density and compromised bone strength. The inhibition of osteoblast activity contributes to the negative impact of cortisol on bone health.

Calcium Regulation:

Cortisol plays a role in calcium homeostasis, influencing the balance of this vital mineral in the body. It can increase urinary calcium excretion, potentially leading to decreased calcium availability for bone formation. Inadequate calcium availability can compromise bone health and increase the risk of osteoporosis.

Impact on Hormones:

Cortisol interacts with other hormones that regulate bone metabolism, such as estrogen and parathyroid hormone (PTH). Imbalances in these hormonal systems, often associated with chronic stress and cortisol dysregulation, can further contribute to bone loss, and increase osteoporosis risk.

Cortisol, Chronic Stress, and Osteoporosis Risk:

Chronic stress and prolonged cortisol elevation can have significant implications for bone health and osteoporosis risk. Here are some key considerations:

Hormonal Imbalances:

Chronic stress and cortisol dysregulation can disrupt the balance of other hormones that influence bone health, such as estrogen and PTH. Reduced estrogen levels, commonly seen in postmenopausal women or individuals with hormonal imbalances, can accelerate bone loss. Similarly, elevated PTH levels can stimulate bone resorption, further exacerbating bone density loss.

Inflammatory Response:

Chronic stress and high cortisol levels can contribute to a chronic low-grade inflammatory state in the body. This inflammatory response can lead to increased bone resorption and interfere with the bone remodeling process, increasing the risk of osteoporosis.

Lifestyle Factors:

Chronic stress and cortisol dysregulation can impact lifestyle factors that contribute to osteoporosis risk. Individuals experiencing chronic stress may engage in unhealthy coping mechanisms such as smoking, excessive ... consumption, or poor dietary choices, all of which can further compromise bone health.

Managing Cortisol for Optimal Bone Health:

To promote optimal bone health and reduce osteoporosis risk, consider the following strategies for managing cortisol levels and mitigating the impact of chronic stress:

Stress Reduction Techniques:

Engage in stress reduction techniques such as mindfulness meditation, deep breathing exercises, yoga, or engaging hobbies. These practices help modulate the stress response, lower cortisol levels, and promote a sense of calm and relaxation.

Physical Activity:

Regular weight-bearing exercises, such as walking, jogging, dancing, or weightlifting, can improve bone density and strength. Engaging in physical activity helps stimulate bone formation and counteract the negative effects of cortisol on bone health.

Nutritional Support:

Ensure an adequate intake of bone-healthy nutrients, including calcium, vitamin D, magnesium, and vitamin K. These nutrients play essential roles in bone metabolism and can support optimal bone health. Consult with a healthcare professional or registered dietitian for personalized dietary recommendations.

Hormone Balance:

Maintain hormone balance, particularly in women approaching menopause or individuals with hormonal imbalances. Consult with a healthcare professional to discuss potential hormone therapies or lifestyle interventions that can support hormonal balance and optimize bone health.

Lifestyle Modifications:

Make lifestyle modifications that promote overall well-being and stress reduction. Prioritize adequate sleep, a balanced diet, smoking cessation, moderation in ... consumption, and healthy coping strategies to minimize chronic stress and cortisol dysregulation.

So,

Cortisol, the stress hormone, has a significant impact on bone health and osteoporosis risk. Elevated cortisol levels can promote bone resorption, inhibit bone formation, and disrupt calcium regulation, leading to reduced bone mineral density and increased susceptibility to osteoporosis.

By managing cortisol levels through stress reduction techniques, regular physical activity, nutritional support, hormone balance, and lifestyle modifications, individuals can support optimal bone health and reduce the risk of osteoporosis. It is essential to adopt a holistic approach to bone health, taking into account the interplay between cortisol, lifestyle factors, hormonal balance, and overall well-being.

Remember, bone health is a lifelong endeavor, and it's never too early or too late to prioritize healthy habits. By managing cortisol and promoting optimal bone health, individuals can safeguard their skeletal well-being and maintain strength and resilience throughout their lives.

Chapter 17: What is the role of cortisol in regulating blood sugar levels?

We will explore the fascinating role of cortisol, the "stress hormone," in regulating blood sugar levels. Cortisol plays a crucial role in our body's stress response and various physiological processes. One of its essential functions is to regulate blood sugar levels, ensuring a steady supply of energy to meet the body's demands. In this chapter, we will delve into the details of how cortisol influences blood sugar regulation, shedding light on the mechanisms involved and offering insights into maintaining a healthy balance for overall well-being.

Understanding Blood Sugar Regulation:

Before we delve into the specifics of cortisol and blood sugar regulation, let's establish a foundational understanding of how blood sugar is regulated in the body. Blood sugar, or glucose, is the primary source of energy for our cells. To maintain a stable blood sugar level, several hormones, and processes work in harmony:

Insulin:

Insulin, produced by the pancreas, helps lower blood sugar levels by facilitating the uptake of glucose into cells. It promotes the storage of excess glucose in the liver and muscles for future energy needs.

Glucagon:

Glucagon, also produced by the pancreas, has the opposite effect of insulin. It raises blood sugar levels by stimulating the breakdown of stored glycogen in the liver, releasing glucose into the bloodstream.

Liver and Muscles:

The liver and muscles store glycogen, a form of glucose that can be readily converted into energy when needed. They play a crucial role in regulating blood sugar levels by releasing or storing glucose based on the body's energy requirements.

Cortisol and Blood Sugar Regulation:

Cortisol influences blood sugar regulation through various mechanisms. Here's how cortisol impacts blood sugar levels:

Glucose Production:

Cortisol stimulates the liver to produce glucose through a process called gluconeogenesis. Gluconeogenesis involves converting non-carbohydrate sources, such as amino acids and glycerol, into glucose. This process increases blood sugar levels and provides an additional energy source during periods of stress or fasting.

Insulin Resistance:

Elevated cortisol levels can contribute to insulin resistance, a condition where the body's cells become less responsive to the effects of insulin. Insulin resistance impairs the ability of insulin to facilitate the uptake of glucose into cells, leading to higher blood sugar levels. Prolonged cortisol elevation and insulin resistance may increase the risk of developing type 2 diabetes.

Counterregulatory Hormone:

Cortisol acts as a counterregulatory hormone, opposing the actions of insulin. During stressful situations or times of increased energy demand, cortisol levels rise, and its actions suppress the effects of insulin, promoting the release of glucose into the bloodstream.

Glucagon Regulation:

Cortisol can influence the release of glucagon, the hormone that raises blood sugar levels. In certain situations, cortisol can enhance the effects of glucagon, leading to increased glucose production and release from the liver.

Cortisol, Stress, and Blood Sugar Dysregulation:

Chronic stress and prolonged cortisol elevation can disrupt blood sugar regulation, potentially leading to blood sugar dysregulation and an increased risk of developing conditions such as insulin resistance and type 2 diabetes. Here are some key considerations:

Gluconeogenesis Imbalance:

Excessive cortisol levels can result in an overactive gluconeogenesis process, leading to elevated blood sugar levels even when glucose is not required for immediate energy needs. This imbalance can contribute to hyperglycemia and impaired blood sugar regulation.

Central Obesity:

Chronic stress and cortisol dysregulation can contribute to central obesity, the accumulation of fat around the abdomen. Central obesity is associated with an increased risk of insulin resistance and metabolic syndrome, both of which can disrupt blood sugar regulation.

Disrupted Insulin Signaling:

Elevated cortisol levels can interfere with the signaling pathways involved in insulin action, impairing the ability of cells to respond to insulin's glucose-lowering effects. This disruption contributes to insulin resistance and elevated blood sugar levels.

Managing Cortisol and Blood Sugar Regulation:

Maintaining a healthy balance in cortisol levels is crucial for optimal blood sugar regulation and overall well-being. Here are some strategies to manage cortisol and support blood sugar balance:

Stress Reduction Techniques:

Engage in stress reduction techniques such as mindfulness meditation, deep breathing exercises, yoga, or engaging hobbies. These practices help modulate the stress response, lower cortisol levels, and promote a sense of calm and relaxation.

Regular Physical Activity:

Incorporate regular physical activity into your routine. Exercise helps regulate cortisol levels and improves insulin sensitivity, supporting optimal blood sugar regulation. Aim for a combination of aerobic exercise, strength training, and flexibility exercises for a comprehensive approach.

Balanced Diet:

Adopt a balanced diet that includes a variety of nutrient-dense foods, such as fruits, vegetables, whole grains, lean proteins, and healthy fats. Avoid excessive intake of sugary and processed foods, as they can contribute to blood sugar dysregulation. Incorporate high-fiber foods to promote steady blood sugar levels.

Adequate Sleep:

Prioritize adequate sleep to support cortisol regulation and overall metabolic health. Aim for 7-9 hours of quality sleep each night, as sleep deprivation and poor sleep quality can disrupt cortisol balance and affect blood sugar regulation.

Lifestyle Modifications:

Make lifestyle modifications that promote overall well-being and stress reduction. Engage in activities that bring joy and relaxation, foster social connections, and promote a healthy work-life balance. Prioritize self-care and engage in activities that help you unwind and manage stress effectively.

So,

Cortisol, the stress hormone, plays a vital role in blood sugar regulation. Elevated cortisol levels can influence blood sugar levels through various mechanisms, including gluconeogenesis stimulation, insulin resistance, counterregulatory effects, and glucagon regulation. Chronic stress and prolonged cortisol elevation can disrupt blood sugar regulation, potentially leading to blood sugar dysregulation and an increased risk of developing conditions such as insulin resistance and type 2 diabetes.

By managing cortisol levels through stress reduction techniques, regular physical activity, a balanced diet, adequate sleep, and lifestyle modifications, individuals can support optimal blood sugar regulation and reduce the risk of developing blood sugar-related conditions. It is essential to adopt a holistic approach to managing cortisol and promoting blood sugar balance, taking into account the interplay between stress, lifestyle factors, and overall well-being.

Remember, maintaining a healthy balance in cortisol levels is a lifelong endeavor. By implementing strategies to manage cortisol and support blood sugar regulation, individuals can empower themselves to lead a healthy and balanced life. Consult with healthcare professionals, such as endocrinologists or registered dietitians, for personalized guidance and recommendations tailored to your specific needs. With mindful attention to cortisol and blood sugar regulation, you can optimize your overall health and well-being.

Chapter 18: Can cortisol levels be influenced by certain medications?

We will explore the intriguing relationship between certain medications and cortisol levels. Cortisol, the "stress hormone," plays a crucial role in our body's stress response and various physiological processes. Medications, whether prescribed or over the counter, can have profound effects on our hormonal balance. In this chapter, we will delve into the details of how certain medications can influence cortisol levels, shedding light on the mechanisms involved and offering insights into understanding and managing medication-related effects on cortisol.

Understanding Cortisol and its Role in the Body:

Before we dive into the specifics of medication effects on cortisol, let's establish a foundational understanding of cortisol and its role in the body. Cortisol is a hormone produced by the adrenal glands in response to stress. It regulates a wide range of physiological processes, including metabolism, immune function, and the body's stress response.

Cortisol Metabolism and Clearance:

Cortisol is metabolized and cleared from the body through various pathways, primarily involving the liver and kidneys. The enzymes involved in cortisol metabolism, such as 11-beta-hydroxysteroid dehydrogenase (11β-HSD), play a critical role in maintaining cortisol balance. Any disruption in these pathways can affect cortisol levels.

Medications and Cortisol Levels:

Several medications have been found to influence cortisol levels through various mechanisms. Here's a closer look at how certain medications can impact cortisol:

Glucocorticoid Medications:

Glucocorticoids, such as prednisone or dexamethasone, are synthetic forms of cortisol commonly prescribed to suppress inflammation and modulate the immune response. These medications mimic the effects of cortisol and can significantly increase cortisol levels when taken orally, intravenously, or through other routes.

Prolonged use of high-dose glucocorticoids can suppress the body's natural cortisol production, leading to adrenal insufficiency when the medication is discontinued.

Exogenous Corticosteroids:

Similar to glucocorticoids, exogenous corticosteroids can influence cortisol levels. These medications, such as hydrocortisone creams or nasal sprays, are often used for their anti-inflammatory properties. When applied topically or locally, their systemic absorption is minimal, and their impact on cortisol levels is generally negligible. However, with long-term or high-dose use, systemic effects can occur, potentially affecting cortisol levels.

Birth Control Pills:

Oral contraceptives, commonly known as birth control pills, contain synthetic hormones, including estrogen and progestin. These hormones can affect cortisol metabolism and clearance. Estrogen, for instance, can increase cortisol-binding globulin (CBG) levels, leading to higher total cortisol levels but potentially lower free cortisol levels. Progestin, on the other hand, can influence cortisol clearance rates. The impact of birth control pills on cortisol levels may vary depending on the specific formulation and individual factors.

Antidepressants:

Certain antidepressant medications, such as selective serotonin reuptake inhibitors (SSRIs), serotonin-norepinephrine reuptake inhibitors (SNRIs), or tricyclic antidepressants (TCAs), can modulate cortisol levels. The exact mechanisms are not fully understood, but these medications may influence cortisol metabolism or interact with the hypothalamic-pituitary-adrenal (HPA) axis, which regulates cortisol production.

Steroid-Based Medications:

Other steroid-based medications, such as anabolic steroids or corticosteroid creams used for skin conditions, may impact cortisol levels. Anabolic steroids, often used illicitly for performance-enhancing purposes, can suppress the body's natural cortisol production, leading to adrenal suppression. Corticosteroid creams, when used topically, usually have minimal systemic absorption, and typically do not significantly affect cortisol levels.

Managing Medication Effects on Cortisol:

If you are taking medications that may influence cortisol levels, it is crucial to be aware of potential effects and work closely with your healthcare provider to monitor and manage cortisol balance. Here are some considerations:

Communication with Healthcare Provider:

Inform your healthcare provider about all the medications you are taking, including prescription drugs, over-the-counter medications, supplements, and herbal remedies. This information helps them assess potential interactions or effects on cortisol levels.

Individualized Monitoring:

If you are prescribed medications known to impact cortisol levels, your healthcare provider may monitor your cortisol levels through blood tests or other assessments. This monitoring helps ensure that cortisol remains within the desired range and provides insights into the medication's impact on your hormonal balance.

Dosage Adjustments:

In some cases, your healthcare provider may need to adjust the dosage or formulation of medications to optimize cortisol balance. This may involve tapering off glucocorticoids, modifying birth control pill formulations, or exploring alternative medications with fewer cortisol-related effects.

Lifestyle Factors:

Adopting healthy lifestyle practices can support cortisol balance alongside medication management. Focus on stress reduction techniques, regular physical activity, adequate sleep, and a balanced diet. These lifestyle factors contribute to overall well-being and can complement medication management.

Open Dialogue:

Maintain open communication with your healthcare provider and raise any concerns or questions you have regarding medication effects on cortisol. Your healthcare team can provide guidance, address any uncertainties, and work collaboratively with you to optimize your treatment plan.

So,

Certain medications can influence cortisol levels through various mechanisms, including direct cortisol supplementation, modulation of cortisol metabolism, or interactions with the HPA axis. Understanding the potential effects of medications on cortisol is important for managing hormonal balance and optimizing treatment outcomes.

If you are taking medications known to impact cortisol levels, it is essential to communicate with your healthcare provider, monitor cortisol levels when necessary, and consider lifestyle factors that support cortisol balance. With informed management and open dialogue with your healthcare team, you can navigate medication-related effects on cortisol and promote overall well-being.

Chapter 19: The Impact of Cortisol on Skin Health and Aging

We will explore the fascinating relationship between cortisol and skin health and aging. Cortisol, commonly known as the "stress hormone," plays a crucial role in our body's stress response and various physiological processes. While cortisol is essential for our well-being, prolonged or excessive cortisol elevation can have implications for skin health and the aging process. In this chapter, we will delve into the details of how cortisol impacts skin health and aging, shedding light on the mechanisms involved and offering insights into maintaining a healthy and vibrant complexion.

Understanding Cortisol and its Role in the Body:

Before we delve into the specifics of cortisol and skin health, let's establish a foundational understanding of cortisol and its role in the body. Cortisol is a hormone produced by the adrenal glands in response to stress. It helps regulate metabolism, immune function, inflammation, and the body's stress response.

The Impact of Cortisol on Skin Health:

Cortisol can influence skin health through various mechanisms. Here's a closer look at how cortisol impacts our skin:

Inflammation and Skin Conditions:

Excessive cortisol levels can contribute to chronic inflammation, which may manifest as skin conditions such as acne, eczema, psoriasis, or rosacea. Inflammation triggers an immune response in the skin, leading to redness, swelling, and irritation.

Impaired Barrier Function:

Cortisol can disrupt the skin's natural barrier function, which is crucial for maintaining hydration and protecting against external aggressors. Elevated cortisol levels can compromise the skin's barrier integrity, resulting in increased water loss, dryness, and heightened sensitivity.

Collagen Breakdown:

Cortisol can contribute to the breakdown of collagen, a protein that provides structural support and elasticity to the skin.

Excessive cortisol exposure can activate enzymes that degrade collagen fibers, leading to a loss of skin firmness, fine lines, and wrinkles.

Delayed Wound Healing:

Elevated cortisol levels can impair the skin's ability to heal wounds efficiently. Cortisol interferes with the inflammatory response necessary for wound repair, potentially delaying the healing process and increasing the risk of scarring.

Skin Aging:

Prolonged cortisol elevation can accelerate the aging process of the skin. Cortisol-induced collagen breakdown, impaired barrier function, and chronic inflammation can contribute to the development of wrinkles, sagging skin, uneven tone, and a dull complexion.

Managing Cortisol for Skin Health:

Maintaining a healthy balance in cortisol levels is crucial for optimal skin health and delaying the signs of aging. Here are some strategies to manage cortisol and support vibrant skin:

Stress Reduction Techniques:

Engage in stress reduction techniques such as meditation, deep breathing exercises, yoga, or mindfulness practices. These activities help modulate the stress response, lower cortisol levels, and promote a sense of calm and relaxation.

Adequate Sleep:

Prioritize quality sleep to support cortisol regulation and overall skin health. During deep sleep, the body undergoes repair and rejuvenation processes, supporting the skin's natural healing mechanisms and preventing premature aging.

Balanced Diet:

Adopt a balanced diet rich in fruits, vegetables, whole grains, lean proteins, and healthy fats. Antioxidant-rich foods, such as berries, leafy greens, and nuts, can help counteract the effects of oxidative stress and inflammation on the skin. Avoid excessive intake of sugary and processed foods, as they can contribute to inflammation and skin damage.

Skincare Routine:

Establish a skincare routine that focuses on gentle cleansing, moisturizing, and sun protection. Choose skincare products formulated with ingredients that support skin health, such as hyaluronic acid for hydration, antioxidants for protection against free radicals, and ceramides to enhance the skin's barrier function.

Sun Protection:

Protect your skin from harmful UV rays by wearing sunscreen with broad-spectrum protection and a sun protection factor (SPF) of 30 or higher. Sun exposure can trigger cortisol release and accelerate skin aging. Additionally, seek shade, wear protective clothing, and avoid excessive sun exposure, especially during peak hours.

Healthy Lifestyle Habits:

Adopting a healthy lifestyle can support overall well-being and vibrant skin. Engage in regular physical activity, which can help manage stress and improve circulation, promoting a healthy complexion. Avoid smoking and limit ... consumption, as these habits can contribute to inflammation and skin damage.

So,

Cortisol, the stress hormone, can have a significant impact on skin health and the aging process. Excessive cortisol levels can contribute to inflammation, impaired barrier function, collagen breakdown, delayed wound healing, and premature skin aging. However, by managing cortisol through stress reduction techniques, adequate sleep, a balanced diet, a skincare routine, sun protection, and healthy lifestyle habits, individuals can support optimal skin health and delay the signs of aging.

Remember, healthy skin reflects overall well-being. By adopting strategies to manage cortisol and prioritize self-care, you can maintain a healthy and vibrant complexion. Consult with dermatologists or skincare professionals for personalized guidance and recommendations tailored to your specific skin concerns. With mindful attention to cortisol and skin health, you can nurture your skin's natural beauty and radiance.

Chapter 20: The Role of Cortisol in the Development and Progression of Cardiovascular Diseases

We will explore the intriguing relationship between cortisol and cardiovascular diseases. Cortisol, commonly known as the "stress hormone," plays a crucial role in our body's stress response and various physiological processes. While cortisol is essential for our well-being, prolonged or excessive cortisol elevation can have implications for cardiovascular health. In this chapter, we will delve into the details of how cortisol impacts the development and progression of cardiovascular diseases, shedding light on the mechanisms involved and offering insights into maintaining a healthy cardiovascular system.

Understanding Cortisol and its Role in the Body:

Before we delve into the specifics of cortisol and cardiovascular diseases, let's establish a foundational understanding of cortisol and its role in the body. Cortisol is a hormone produced by the adrenal glands in response to stress. It helps regulate metabolism, immune function, inflammation, and the body's stress response.

Cortisol and Cardiovascular Health:

Cortisol can influence cardiovascular health through various mechanisms. Here's a closer look at how cortisol impacts our cardiovascular system:

Blood Pressure Regulation:

Cortisol plays a role in blood pressure regulation by affecting the function of blood vessels and the renin-angiotensin-aldosterone system. Elevated cortisol levels can contribute to vasoconstriction, narrowing of blood vessels, and increased blood pressure. Prolonged hypertension can lead to the development and progression of cardiovascular diseases.

Inflammation and Atherosclerosis:

Chronic inflammation is a key contributor to the development of atherosclerosis, a condition characterized by the accumulation of plaque in the arteries. Cortisol, when excessively elevated, can promote inflammation and contribute to the progression of atherosclerosis, potentially leading to conditions such as coronary artery disease.

Lipid Metabolism:

Cortisol can impact lipid metabolism, influencing the levels of cholesterol and triglycerides in the bloodstream. Elevated cortisol levels can lead to increased production of triglycerides and a redistribution of fat storage, favoring the accumulation of visceral fat. These lipid abnormalities can contribute to the development of cardiovascular diseases.

Insulin Resistance:

Prolonged cortisol elevation can contribute to insulin resistance, a condition where the body's cells become less responsive to the effects of insulin. Insulin resistance can lead to the development of metabolic syndrome, a cluster of conditions that increase the risk of cardiovascular diseases, including hypertension, dyslipidemia, and type 2 diabetes.

Platelet Aggregation:

Cortisol can influence platelet aggregation, the process by which platelets clump together to form blood clots. Excessive cortisol levels can promote platelet aggregation, potentially increasing the risk of clot formation and cardiovascular events such as heart attacks or strokes.

Managing Cortisol for Cardiovascular Health:

Maintaining a healthy balance in cortisol levels is crucial for optimal cardiovascular health. Here are some strategies to manage cortisol and support a healthy cardiovascular system:

Stress Reduction Techniques:

Engage in stress reduction techniques such as meditation, deep breathing exercises, yoga, or mindfulness practices. These activities help modulate the stress response, lower cortisol levels, and promote a sense of calm and relaxation, supporting cardiovascular health.

Regular Physical Activity:

Incorporate regular physical activity into your routine. Exercise helps manage stress, improve cardiovascular fitness, and promote healthy blood pressure levels. Aim for a combination of aerobic exercises, strength training, and flexibility exercises for a comprehensive approach.

Balanced Diet:

Adopt a balanced diet rich in fruits, vegetables, whole grains, lean proteins, and healthy fats. Reduce the intake of processed foods, saturated fats, and added sugars, as they can contribute to inflammation, dyslipidemia, and cardiovascular risk factors.

Blood Pressure Management:

Monitor and manage blood pressure levels regularly. If necessary, work with healthcare professionals to develop a plan that may include lifestyle modifications, medication, and regular check-ups to ensure optimal blood pressure control.

Healthy Weight Management:

Maintain a healthy weight through a combination of regular physical activity and a balanced diet. Excessive weight, particularly around the waistline, can increase the risk of cardiovascular diseases. Consult with healthcare professionals or registered dietitians for personalized guidance and support.

Smoking Cessation:

If you smoke, take steps to quit smoking. Smoking is a significant risk factor for cardiovascular diseases. Seek support from healthcare professionals, join smoking cessation programs, or explore nicotine replacement therapies to improve cardiovascular health.

So,

Cortisol, the stress hormone, can have a significant impact on cardiovascular health. Prolonged or excessive cortisol elevation can contribute to hypertension, chronic inflammation, dyslipidemia, insulin resistance, and platelet aggregation, all of which are risk factors for cardiovascular diseases.

By managing cortisol through stress reduction techniques, regular physical activity, a balanced diet, blood pressure management, healthy weight management, and smoking cessation, individuals can support optimal cardiovascular health. It is important to work closely with healthcare professionals to monitor cardiovascular risk factors, receive appropriate screenings, and address any concerns or symptoms related to cardiovascular health.

Remember, maintaining a healthy cardiovascular system is a lifelong endeavor. By adopting strategies to manage cortisol and prioritize cardiovascular health, individuals can reduce the risk of developing cardiovascular diseases and promote overall well-being. Consult with healthcare professionals, such as cardiologists or primary care physicians, for personalized guidance and recommendations tailored to your specific needs. With mindful attention to cortisol and cardiovascular health, you can nurture a strong and resilient cardiovascular system for a long and healthy life.

Chapter 21: The Interplay of Cortisol with Other Hormones in the Body

We will explore the intricate dance of hormones in our body and specifically focus on the interplay between cortisol, the "stress hormone," and other hormones. Hormones are chemical messengers that regulate various physiological processes and work in harmony to maintain balance and homeostasis. Cortisol, produced by the adrenal glands, interacts with numerous hormones, influencing their production, release, and effects. In this chapter, we will delve into the details of how cortisol interacts with other hormones, shedding light on the mechanisms involved and offering insights into the intricate hormonal symphony within our bodies.

Understanding Hormones and their Functions:

Before we delve into the specifics of cortisol's interactions with other hormones, let's establish a foundational understanding of hormones and their functions in the body. Hormones are produced by various glands and tissues and are released into the bloodstream to act on specific target cells or organs. They play a vital role in regulating growth, metabolism, reproduction, mood, and numerous other physiological processes.

Cortisol and its Role in Hormonal Interactions:

Cortisol, a steroid hormone, interacts with several other hormones, either directly or indirectly, to orchestrate various physiological responses. Here's a closer look at some of the key interactions between cortisol and other hormones:

Hypothalamic-Pituitary-Adrenal (HPA) Axis:

The HPA axis is a complex hormonal system involved in the regulation of cortisol production. The hypothalamus releases corticotropin-releasing hormone (CRH), which stimulates the pituitary gland to produce adrenocorticotropic hormone (ACTH). ACTH, in turn, signals the adrenal glands to release cortisol. Feedback mechanisms ensure that cortisol levels remain within the desired range, with cortisol providing negative feedback to suppress the release of CRH and ACTH.

Growth Hormone (GH):

Cortisol can influence the production and release of growth hormone. Excessive cortisol levels can suppress growth hormone secretion, potentially leading to growth impairment in children and decreased muscle mass in adults. On the other hand, growth hormone deficiency can result in increased cortisol levels, as growth hormone helps regulate cortisol metabolism.

Thyroid Hormones:

Cortisol and thyroid hormones have intricate interactions. Cortisol can modulate the conversion of the inactive thyroid hormone, thyroxine (T4), into the active form, triiodothyronine (T3). High cortisol levels can decrease the conversion of T4 to T3, leading to a decrease in thyroid hormone activity. Conversely, low thyroid hormone levels can impact cortisol metabolism and contribute to alterations in the HPA axis.

Insulin:

Cortisol and insulin have complex interactions that influence glucose metabolism. Cortisol can induce insulin resistance, impairing the body's ability to respond to insulin and leading to elevated blood sugar levels. Conversely, insulin can modulate cortisol metabolism and reduce cortisol production.

Sex Hormones:

Cortisol can affect the production and release of sex hormones, including estrogen and testosterone. Prolonged cortisol elevation can disrupt the delicate balance of sex hormone production, potentially leading to menstrual irregularities, reduced fertility, and altered libido. Conversely, sex hormones can influence cortisol metabolism and modulate the stress response.

Managing Hormonal Interactions for Balance:

Maintaining a healthy balance among hormones is crucial for optimal health and well-being. Here are some strategies to support hormonal balance and manage the interactions between cortisol and other hormones:

Stress Reduction Techniques:

Engage in stress reduction techniques such as meditation, deep breathing exercises, yoga, or mindfulness practices. Chronic stress and elevated cortisol levels can disrupt the delicate hormonal balance. By managing stress, cortisol levels can be regulated, allowing other hormones to function optimally.

Balanced Diet:

Adopt a balanced diet rich in nutrient-dense foods to support hormonal balance. Include a variety of fruits, vegetables, whole grains, lean proteins, and healthy fats in your meals. Nutrients such as omega-3 fatty acids, vitamin D, and magnesium are particularly important for hormone production and regulation.

Regular Physical Activity:

Incorporate regular physical activity into your routine. Exercise helps modulate hormone levels, improve insulin sensitivity, and promote overall hormonal balance. Aim for a combination of cardiovascular exercises, strength training, and flexibility exercises for a comprehensive approach.

Sleep and Rest:

Prioritize adequate sleep and rest to support hormonal balance. Lack of sleep can disrupt hormone production and regulation, including cortisol. Aim for 7-9 hours of quality sleep each night and establish a consistent sleep routine.

Hormone Replacement Therapy (HRT):

In some cases, individuals may require hormone replacement therapy to restore hormonal balance. This is commonly used in conditions such as thyroid disorders, menopause, or adrenal insufficiency. Consult with healthcare professionals, such as endocrinologists or gynecologists, for personalized guidance and recommendations.

So,

Cortisol, the stress hormone, interacts with a multitude of other hormones in our body, influencing their production, release, and effects. Maintaining a healthy hormonal balance is crucial for overall health and well-being. By managing cortisol through stress reduction techniques, a balanced diet, regular physical activity, adequate sleep, and seeking appropriate medical interventions, when necessary, individuals can support optimal hormonal balance.

Remember, the interplay between hormones is complex and individualized. It is essential to consult with healthcare professionals, such as endocrinologists or primary care physicians, for personalized guidance and recommendations tailored to your specific hormonal needs. With mindful attention to cortisol and its interactions with other hormones, you can nurture a harmonious hormonal symphony within your body, promoting optimal health and vitality.

Chapter 22: The Relationship between Cortisol and Inflammation

We will explore the intriguing relationship between cortisol and inflammation. Cortisol, commonly known as the "stress hormone," plays a crucial role in our body's stress response and various physiological processes. Inflammation, on the other hand, is a complex biological response that is triggered by the immune system in response to harmful stimuli. In this chapter, we will delve into the details of how cortisol interacts with inflammation, shedding light on the mechanisms involved and offering insights into the intricate relationship between these two processes.

Understanding Inflammation:

Before we delve into the specifics of cortisol and inflammation, let's establish a foundational understanding of inflammation. Inflammation is a vital part of our immune response, aimed at protecting the body from injury, infection, or disease. It involves a series of complex cellular and molecular processes that result in redness, swelling, heat, and pain in the affected area.

Acute vs. Chronic Inflammation:

There are two types of inflammation: acute and chronic. Acute inflammation is a short-term response triggered by an injury or infection. It is a necessary and beneficial process that helps the body heal. On the other hand, chronic inflammation is a persistent and long-lasting response that can be detrimental to health. Chronic inflammation is often associated with underlying conditions such as autoimmune diseases, cardiovascular diseases, and certain cancers.

Cortisol and its Anti-inflammatory Properties:

Cortisol has potent anti-inflammatory properties that help regulate and resolve the inflammatory response. Here's a closer look at how cortisol interacts with inflammation:

Suppression of Immune Response:

Cortisol acts to suppress the immune system, particularly the inflammatory response. It inhibits the production and release of pro-inflammatory cytokines, which are molecules that play a key role in initiating and amplifying the inflammatory process. By dampening the immune response, cortisol helps to control and resolve inflammation.

Inhibition of Inflammatory Mediators:

Cortisol inhibits the synthesis and release of inflammatory mediators, such as prostaglandins and leukotrienes. These molecules are involved in the initiation and propagation of inflammation, promoting vasodilation, swelling, and pain. By reducing their production, cortisol helps to dampen the inflammatory process.

Modulation of Immune Cells:

Cortisol can influence the function of various immune cells involved in the inflammatory response, such as neutrophils, macrophages, and lymphocytes. It can suppress the activation and migration of these cells, leading to a reduction in inflammation.

Control of Transcription Factors:

Cortisol can modulate the activity of transcription factors, which are proteins that regulate gene expression. It interacts with transcription factors such as nuclear factor-kappa B (NF-$\varkappa$B) and activator protein-1 (AP-1), which are critical for the expression of pro-inflammatory genes. By inhibiting the activity of these transcription factors, cortisol helps to downregulate the production of pro-inflammatory proteins.

Managing Cortisol and Inflammation for Health:

Maintaining a balance between cortisol and inflammation is crucial for optimal health. Here are some strategies to manage cortisol and inflammation:

Stress Reduction Techniques:

Engage in stress reduction techniques such as meditation, deep breathing exercises, yoga, or mindfulness practices. Chronic stress can lead to dysregulation of cortisol levels and contribute to chronic inflammation. By managing stress, cortisol levels can be regulated, supporting a healthy inflammatory response.

Regular Physical Activity:

Incorporate regular physical activity into your routine. Exercise has anti-inflammatory effects and helps regulate cortisol levels. Aim for a combination of cardiovascular exercises, strength training, and flexibility exercises for a comprehensive approach.

Balanced Diet:

Adopt a balanced diet rich in fruits, vegetables, whole grains, lean proteins, and healthy fats. Include foods with anti-inflammatory properties, such as fatty fish, turmeric, ginger, and green leafy vegetables. Avoid excessive consumption of processed foods, sugary beverages, and trans fats, as they can contribute to inflammation.

Adequate Sleep:

Prioritize quality sleep to support cortisol regulation and overall health. Lack of sleep can contribute to chronic inflammation and dysregulation of cortisol levels. Aim for 7-9 hours of quality sleep each night and establish a consistent sleep routine.

Mindful Approach to Health:

Adopt a mindful approach to your overall health. Take care of your mental and emotional well-being through practices such as mindfulness meditation, therapy, or engaging in hobbies and activities that bring joy and relaxation. Managing chronic stress and promoting emotional well-being can positively influence cortisol levels and support a healthy inflammatory response.

Consultation with Healthcare Professionals:

If you have chronic inflammation or suspect imbalances in cortisol levels, consult with healthcare professionals, such as rheumatologists, immunologists, or endocrinologists. They can provide a comprehensive evaluation, diagnose underlying conditions, and develop a tailored treatment plan.

So,

Cortisol, the stress hormone, plays a vital role in the regulation of inflammation. Through its anti-inflammatory properties, cortisol helps to suppress the immune response, inhibit the production of inflammatory mediators, modulate immune cell function, and control transcription factors involved in inflammation. Maintaining a healthy balance between cortisol and inflammation is essential for optimal health and well-being.

By adopting strategies to manage cortisol and support a healthy inflammatory response through stress reduction techniques, regular physical activity, a balanced diet, adequate sleep, and a mindful approach to health, individuals can promote a healthy balance between cortisol and inflammation.

Remember, chronic inflammation can be detrimental to health and contribute to the development and progression of various diseases. If you have concerns about chronic inflammation or imbalances in cortisol levels, consult with healthcare professionals who can provide guidance, conduct appropriate evaluations, and develop a personalized treatment plan.

With mindful attention to cortisol and its interactions with inflammation, you can nurture a harmonious relationship within your body, promoting optimal health and well-being.

Chapter 23: The Impact of Environmental Toxins on Cortisol Levels

We will explore the intriguing relationship between environmental toxins and cortisol levels. Cortisol, commonly known as the "stress hormone," plays a crucial role in our body's stress response and various physiological processes. Environmental toxins, on the other hand, are substances present in our surroundings that can have harmful effects on our health. In this chapter, we will delve into the details of how exposure to environmental toxins can impact cortisol levels, shedding light on the mechanisms involved and offering insights into understanding and managing the effects of toxins on cortisol.

Understanding Environmental Toxins:

Before we delve into the specifics of environmental toxins and cortisol, let's establish a foundational understanding of environmental toxins. Environmental toxins are substances found in our environment that have the potential to cause harm to human health. They can come from various sources such as air pollution, water contamination, pesticides, heavy metals, industrial chemicals, and household products.

Impact of Environmental Toxins on Cortisol Levels:

Exposure to environmental toxins can influence cortisol levels through various mechanisms. Here's a closer look at how environmental toxins can impact cortisol:

Disruption of Hormonal Pathways:

Some environmental toxins have the potential to disrupt the delicate balance of hormones in our body, including cortisol. For example, certain chemicals found in pesticides, industrial pollutants, and endocrine-disrupting substances can interfere with the normal functioning of the hypothalamic-pituitary-adrenal (HPA) axis, which regulates cortisol production. This disruption can lead to dysregulation of cortisol levels.

Oxidative Stress:

Many environmental toxins induce oxidative stress, a condition characterized by an imbalance between the production of free radicals and the body's ability to counteract their harmful effects.

Oxidative stress can trigger an inflammatory response and impact the HPA axis, potentially leading to alterations in cortisol production and release.

Neurotoxicity:

Certain environmental toxins, such as heavy metals (e.g., lead, mercury) and some industrial chemicals, can exert neurotoxic effects. The nervous system, including the brain regions involved in regulating the stress response, can be affected by these toxins. Disruption of neural pathways involved in cortisol regulation can lead to abnormal cortisol levels.

Immune Activation:

Exposure to certain environmental toxins, such as air pollutants and particulate matter, can activate the immune system. Inflammatory responses triggered by immune activation can impact the HPA axis and cortisol production. Chronic exposure to air pollution, for example, has been associated with alterations in cortisol levels.

Managing Exposure to Environmental Toxins and Cortisol Levels:

While we cannot completely eliminate our exposure to environmental toxins, there are strategies to minimize their impact on cortisol levels and overall health. Here are some approaches to consider:

Environmental Awareness:

Stay informed about potential sources of environmental toxins and take steps to minimize exposure. This includes avoiding or minimizing contact with known pollutants, using household and personal care products that are free from harmful chemicals, and ensuring proper ventilation in indoor spaces.

Nutrient-Rich Diet:

Adopt a nutrient-rich diet that supports the body's natural detoxification processes. Include foods rich in antioxidants, such as fruits, vegetables, nuts, and seeds. Antioxidants help counteract the harmful effects of free radicals generated by environmental toxins, thereby reducing oxidative stress.

Regular Physical Activity:

Engage in regular physical activity to support overall health and promote detoxification. Exercise stimulates blood circulation, lymphatic flow, and sweating, which aid in the elimination of toxins from the body. However, be mindful of potential exposure to outdoor pollutants during exercise and choose clean and well-ventilated environments whenever possible.

Indoor Air Quality:

Improve indoor air quality by minimizing the use of chemical-based products, ensuring proper ventilation, and using air purifiers if necessary. Regularly clean and dust your living space to reduce the accumulation of environmental toxins, especially in carpets, furniture, and household appliances.

Water Filtration:

Invest in a water filtration system to reduce exposure to contaminants in tap water. Choose a filtration system that effectively removes common toxins, such as heavy metals, pesticides, and industrial chemicals.

Consultation with Healthcare Professionals:

If you suspect exposure to environmental toxins or have concerns about cortisol levels, consult with healthcare professionals who specialize in environmental medicine or toxicology. They can provide guidance, conduct appropriate evaluations, and develop a personalized treatment plan.

So,

Exposure to environmental toxins can impact cortisol levels through various mechanisms, including disruption of hormonal pathways, oxidative stress, neurotoxicity, and immune activation. While complete avoidance of environmental toxins may be challenging, adopting strategies to minimize exposure, supporting detoxification processes through a nutrient-rich diet, regular physical activity, and improving indoor air and water quality can help reduce the impact on cortisol levels and overall health.

Remember, it is important to stay informed, take proactive steps to reduce exposure to environmental toxins, and seek professional guidance when necessary. By minimizing exposure and supporting the body's natural detoxification processes, you can optimize cortisol levels and promote overall well-being. Furthermore, promoting environmental sustainability and advocating for policies that protect against environmental toxins can contribute to a healthier and safer living environment for everyone. Together, we can work towards creating a world that supports optimal health and well-being while minimizing the risks associated with environmental toxins and their impact on cortisol and other vital physiological processes.

Chapter 24: The Influence of Cortisol on Hair Growth and Loss

We will explore the intriguing relationship between cortisol and hair growth and loss. Cortisol, commonly known as the "stress hormone," plays a crucial role in our body's stress response and various physiological processes. Hair growth and loss, on the other hand, are dynamic processes influenced by a combination of genetic, hormonal, and environmental factors. In this chapter, we will delve into the details of how cortisol interacts with hair growth and loss, shedding light on the mechanisms involved and offering insights into understanding and managing the effects of cortisol on our locks.

Understanding Hair Growth and Loss:

Before we delve into the specifics of cortisol and its impact on hair, let's establish a foundational understanding of hair growth and loss. Hair growth occurs in cycles, with each hair follicle going through a growth phase (anagen), a transitional phase (catagen), and a resting phase (telogen). Shedding of hair is a normal part of the hair cycle, with new hair replacing the old. However, various factors can disrupt this delicate balance, leading to excessive hair loss or impaired hair growth.

Cortisol and Hair Growth:

Cortisol can influence hair growth through several mechanisms. Here's a closer look at how cortisol impacts our locks:

Telogen Effluvium:

Prolonged or excessive cortisol elevation can lead to a condition called telogen effluvium, which is characterized by excessive hair shedding. In response to stress or hormonal imbalances, more hair follicles enter the resting phase (telogen) prematurely, resulting in noticeable hair loss. This condition is usually temporary, and hair growth resumes once the underlying stressor is resolved.

Impaired Hair Follicle Function:

Elevated cortisol levels can disrupt the normal functioning of hair follicles. Cortisol-induced oxidative stress and inflammation can damage hair follicles and impede their ability to produce healthy hair. This can result in thinning, brittle hair and a slowed rate of hair growth.

Hormonal Imbalances:

Cortisol interacts with other hormones in the body, such as sex hormones and thyroid hormones, which can also impact hair growth. Hormonal imbalances, including elevated cortisol levels, can disrupt the delicate balance necessary for healthy hair growth. For example, excessive cortisol levels can contribute to the suppression of sex hormone production, leading to changes in hair texture, thickness, and overall hair quality.

Managing Cortisol for Healthy Hair:

Maintaining a healthy balance in cortisol levels is crucial for promoting optimal hair growth and minimizing hair loss. Here are some strategies to manage cortisol and support healthy hair:

Stress Reduction Techniques:

Engage in stress reduction techniques such as meditation, deep breathing exercises, yoga, or mindfulness practices. Chronic stress can lead to dysregulation of cortisol levels, which can negatively impact hair growth. By managing stress, cortisol levels can be regulated, supporting healthy hair growth.

Balanced Diet:

Adopt a balanced diet rich in nutrients that support hair health. Include a variety of fruits, vegetables, whole grains, lean proteins, and healthy fats. Nutrients such as vitamins A, C, E, biotin, zinc, and omega-3 fatty acids are particularly important for promoting hair growth and maintaining its strength and luster.

Scalp Care:

Maintain a healthy scalp environment by keeping it clean and well-nourished. Gently cleanse the scalp regularly to remove excess sebum, dirt, and product buildup. Use scalp-friendly hair care products that do not contain harsh chemicals or irritants. Massaging the scalp can also stimulate blood flow to the hair follicles and promote healthy hair growth.

Avoid Excessive Heat and Chemical Treatments:

Excessive heat from styling tools and harsh chemical treatments can damage hair and weaken its structure. Minimize the use of heat styling tools, use heat protectant products, and opt for gentle and natural hair care routines. Avoid frequent use of chemical treatments such as relaxers, perms, and hair dyes, as they can weaken hair and contribute to breakage.

Hair-Friendly Lifestyle Habits:

Adopt lifestyle habits that promote overall health, which in turn supports healthy hair growth. Get regular physical activity, prioritize quality sleep, stay hydrated, and avoid smoking and excessive ... consumption. These habits contribute to optimal hormonal balance and overall well-being, which can positively impact hair health.

Consultation with Healthcare Professionals:

If you have concerns about hair loss or suspect imbalances in cortisol levels, consult with healthcare professionals who specialize in hair health, such as dermatologists or trichologists. They can provide guidance, evaluate potential underlying causes, and develop a personalized treatment plan.

So,

Cortisol, the stress hormone, can impact hair growth and loss through various mechanisms, including telogen effluvium, impaired hair follicle function, and hormonal imbalances. By managing cortisol through stress reduction techniques, a balanced diet, scalp care, avoidance of excessive heat and chemical treatments, hair-friendly lifestyle habits, and seeking professional guidance, when necessary, individuals can support healthy hair growth and minimize hair loss.

Remember, maintaining healthy hair is a holistic endeavor that involves not only addressing cortisol levels but also considering other factors such as genetics, overall health, and environmental influences. Embrace a comprehensive approach to hair care, prioritize self-care, and consult with professionals for personalized guidance and recommendations. With mindful attention to cortisol and its impact on hair, you can nurture and maintain luscious locks that reflect your inner vitality and well-being.

Chapter 25: The Role of Cortisol in Regulating Blood Pressure

We will explore the fascinating role of cortisol in regulating blood pressure. Cortisol, commonly known as the "stress hormone," is a vital hormone that plays a crucial role in our body's stress response and various physiological processes. Blood pressure, on the other hand, is a fundamental measure of the force exerted by circulating blood against the walls of our blood vessels. In this chapter, we will delve into the details of how cortisol influences blood pressure regulation, shedding light on the mechanisms involved and offering insights into understanding and managing the effects of cortisol on this vital cardiovascular parameter.

Understanding Blood Pressure:

Before we delve into the specifics of cortisol and its role in blood pressure regulation, let's establish a foundational understanding of blood pressure. Blood pressure is measured as two values: systolic pressure (the higher value) and diastolic pressure (the lower value). Systolic pressure represents the force exerted on arterial walls when the heart contracts, while diastolic pressure represents the force when the heart is at rest between beats. Blood pressure is expressed in millimeters of mercury (mmHg) and is measured with a blood pressure cuff and sphygmomanometer.

Cortisol and Blood Pressure Regulation:

Cortisol influences blood pressure through various mechanisms. Here's a closer look at how cortisol impacts blood pressure regulation:

Vascular Tone:

Cortisol affects blood pressure by influencing vascular tone, which refers to the degree of constriction or relaxation of blood vessels. Elevated cortisol levels can lead to vasoconstriction, narrowing of blood vessels, and increased resistance to blood flow. This can result in an increase in blood pressure. Conversely, when cortisol levels decrease, blood vessels can relax, leading to vasodilation and a potential decrease in blood pressure.

Renin-Angiotensin-Aldosterone System (RAAS):

Cortisol interacts with the renin-angiotensin-aldosterone system (RAAS), a complex hormonal system involved in blood pressure regulation. Cortisol can stimulate the release of renin, an enzyme that triggers a cascade of reactions leading to the production of angiotensin II, a potent vasoconstrictor. Angiotensin II promotes the secretion of aldosterone, a hormone that increases sodium and water reabsorption in the kidneys. The retention of sodium and water contributes to an increase in blood volume, which in turn raises blood pressure.

Fluid and Electrolyte Balance:

Cortisol influences blood pressure through its effects on fluid and electrolyte balance. It promotes the reabsorption of sodium by the kidneys and inhibits the reabsorption of potassium. These actions can impact the osmotic balance of body fluids and contribute to alterations in blood pressure.

Stress Response:

Cortisol is a key component of the body's stress response, commonly known as the "fight-or-flight" response. In response to stress, cortisol levels rise, triggering physiological changes that prepare the body for action. These changes include increased heart rate and blood pressure, ensuring adequate blood flow to essential organs and muscles during stressful situations. However, prolonged, or chronic stress can lead to sustained cortisol elevation, which can contribute to chronic hypertension if not properly managed.

Managing Cortisol for Healthy Blood Pressure:

Maintaining a healthy balance in cortisol levels is crucial for optimal blood pressure regulation. Here are some strategies to manage cortisol and support healthy blood pressure:

Stress Reduction Techniques:

Engage in stress reduction techniques such as meditation, deep breathing exercises, yoga, or mindfulness practices. Chronic stress can lead to dysregulation of cortisol levels, potentially contributing to elevated blood pressure. By managing stress, cortisol levels can be regulated, supporting healthy blood pressure.

Regular Physical Activity:

Incorporate regular physical activity into your routine. Exercise has been shown to help regulate cortisol levels and promote cardiovascular health. Aim for a combination of aerobic exercises, strength training, and flexibility exercises for a comprehensive approach. Consult with healthcare professionals for personalized exercise recommendations.

Balanced Diet:

Adopt a balanced diet rich in fruits, vegetables, whole grains, lean proteins, and healthy fats. Reduce the intake of sodium, processed foods, and added sugars, as they can contribute to elevated blood pressure. Include potassium-rich foods such as bananas, avocados, spinach, and sweet potatoes, as potassium helps counterbalance the effects of sodium on blood pressure.

Limit ... and Caffeine Intake:

Limit ... consumption and be mindful of caffeine intake. Excessive ... consumption can raise blood pressure, and caffeine can temporarily elevate blood pressure in some individuals. Moderation is key, and it's important to be aware of how these substances affect your blood pressure.

Maintain a Healthy Weight:

Maintain a healthy weight through a combination of regular physical activity and a balanced diet. Excess weight, particularly around the waistline, can contribute to elevated blood pressure. Consult with healthcare professionals or registered dietitians for personalized guidance and support.

Regular Blood Pressure Monitoring:

Monitor your blood pressure regularly. If you have concerns about your blood pressure or suspect imbalances in cortisol levels, consult with healthcare professionals, such as primary care physicians or cardiologists. They can provide guidance, perform appropriate evaluations, and develop a personalized treatment plan.

So,

Cortisol, the stress hormone, plays a significant role in blood pressure regulation. Through its effects on vascular tone, the renin-angiotensin-aldosterone system, fluid and electrolyte balance, and the body's stress response, cortisol can influence blood pressure levels. By managing cortisol through stress reduction techniques, regular physical activity, a balanced diet, maintaining a healthy weight, and seeking professional guidance, when necessary, individuals can support healthy blood pressure regulation.

Remember, maintaining healthy blood pressure is important for overall cardiovascular health and reducing the risk of conditions such as hypertension. By adopting a holistic approach that encompasses lifestyle modifications, stress management, and regular monitoring, you can support optimal blood pressure levels and promote a healthy cardiovascular system.

Chapter 26: The Influence of Cortisol on the Body's Response to Pain

We will explore the intriguing relationship between cortisol and the body's response to pain. Cortisol, commonly known as the "stress hormone," plays a crucial role in our body's stress response and various physiological processes. Pain, on the other hand, is a complex and subjective experience that can vary in intensity and duration. In this chapter, we will delve into the details of how cortisol influences the body's response to pain, shedding light on the mechanisms involved and offering insights into understanding and managing the effects of cortisol on pain perception.

Understanding Pain:

Before we delve into the specifics of cortisol and pain, let's establish a foundational understanding of pain. Pain is a protective mechanism that alerts us to potential or actual tissue damage. It is a complex experience that involves not only the physical sensation but also emotional and cognitive aspects. Pain can be categorized as acute or chronic, depending on its duration. Acute pain is typically short-lived and serves as a warning signal, while chronic pain persists for an extended period and can be challenging to manage.

Cortisol and Pain Perception:

Cortisol can influence the body's response to pain through various mechanisms. Here's a closer look at how cortisol impacts pain perception:

Anti-inflammatory Effects:

Cortisol has potent anti-inflammatory properties. In the presence of tissue damage or inflammation that contributes to pain, cortisol can suppress the production of pro-inflammatory cytokines and other mediators involved in the inflammatory response. By reducing inflammation, cortisol can indirectly alleviate pain associated with inflammatory conditions.

Modulation of the Stress Response:

Pain and stress share common pathways in the brain and can influence each other. Cortisol, as a key component of the body's stress response, can modulate the body's perception of pain. During stressful situations, cortisol levels rise, and this can affect pain perception. Higher cortisol levels can sometimes lead to a decrease in pain sensitivity, providing a temporary analgesic effect.

Interaction with the Endogenous Opioid System:

Cortisol can interact with the body's endogenous opioid system, which plays a role in pain modulation. Opioids are neurotransmitters that can reduce pain perception by binding to opioid receptors in the brain and spinal cord. Cortisol can influence the production and release of endogenous opioids, potentially affecting pain sensitivity.

Cognitive and Emotional Factors:

Cortisol can influence cognitive and emotional factors that shape the perception and experience of pain. Stress, which can elevate cortisol levels, can amplify the emotional and cognitive components of pain. Negative emotions, such as anxiety and fear, can intensify pain perception, while positive emotions and a relaxed state of mind can have analgesic effects.

Managing Cortisol and Pain Perception:

Maintaining a healthy balance in cortisol levels is crucial for managing pain perception effectively. Here are some strategies to manage cortisol and support a healthier response to pain:

Stress Reduction Techniques:

Engage in stress reduction techniques such as meditation, deep breathing exercises, yoga, or mindfulness practices. Chronic stress can lead to dysregulation of cortisol levels, which can impact pain perception. By managing stress, cortisol levels can be regulated, potentially leading to a more balanced and controlled pain response.

Regular Physical Activity:

Incorporate regular physical activity into your routine. Exercise has been shown to have pain-relieving effects by releasing endorphins, which are natural pain-relieving substances in the body. Consult with healthcare professionals for personalized exercise recommendations, taking into account any existing pain conditions or limitations.

Cognitive Behavioral Therapy:

Consider cognitive behavioral therapy (CBT) as an adjunctive treatment for pain management. CBT focuses on changing thoughts and behaviors related to pain, and it can help individuals develop coping mechanisms and reduce stress. By addressing cognitive and emotional factors associated with pain, CBT can contribute to a healthier pain response.

Pain Medications and Interventions:

In some cases, pain medications or interventions may be necessary to manage pain effectively. Consult with healthcare professionals, such as pain specialists or physicians, who can provide guidance, evaluate the underlying causes of pain, and recommend appropriate treatments. It's important to use pain medications as prescribed and under medical supervision to avoid potential side effects or dependency.

Supportive Lifestyle Factors:

Maintain a healthy lifestyle that supports overall well-being. This includes getting adequate sleep, maintaining a balanced diet, and engaging in activities that promote relaxation and positive emotions. These lifestyle factors can help optimize cortisol levels and support a healthier response to pain.

Consultation with Healthcare Professionals:

If you have chronic or persistent pain, or if you suspect imbalances in cortisol levels, consult with healthcare professionals who specialize in pain management or endocrinology. They can provide a comprehensive evaluation, diagnose underlying conditions, and develop a personalized treatment plan that addresses both the pain and cortisol regulation.

So,

Cortisol, the stress hormone, can influence the body's response to pain through its anti-inflammatory effects, modulation of the stress response, interaction with the endogenous opioid system, and impact on cognitive and emotional factors. By managing cortisol through stress reduction techniques, regular physical activity, cognitive-behavioral therapy, and seeking professional guidance, when necessary, individuals can support a healthier response to pain.

Remember, pain is a multifaceted experience that can be influenced by various factors, including cortisol levels. By adopting a holistic approach that encompasses physical, emotional, and cognitive aspects, individuals can optimize their pain management strategies and work towards a healthier and more balanced pain response.

Chapter 27: The Influence of Gut Health and the Microbiome on Cortisol Levels

We will explore the intriguing relationship between gut health, the microbiome, and cortisol levels. Cortisol, commonly known as the "stress hormone," plays a crucial role in our body's stress response and various physiological processes. The gut, often referred to as our "second brain," and its resident microbial community, known as the microbiome, have emerged as key players in our overall health. In this chapter, we will delve into the details of how gut health and the microbiome can influence cortisol levels, shedding light on the mechanisms involved and offering insights into understanding and managing the effects of these factors on our stress response.

Understanding Gut Health and the Microbiome:

Before we delve into the specifics of gut health, the microbiome, and cortisol, let's establish a foundational understanding of these terms. The gut, or gastrointestinal tract, is a complex system responsible for digesting and absorbing nutrients, as well as playing a vital role in our immune function and overall well-being. The microbiome refers to the trillions of microorganisms, including bacteria, fungi, viruses, and other microbes, that reside in our gut. These microbes have a symbiotic relationship with us, influencing various aspects of our health, including digestion, nutrient absorption, immune function, and even our mental health.

The Gut-Brain Axis and Cortisol Levels:

The gut and the brain are connected through a bidirectional communication system known as the gut-brain axis. This communication occurs via neural, endocrine, and immune pathways, allowing for constant crosstalk between the gut and the brain. Cortisol, as a key hormone involved in the stress response, can be influenced by the gut-brain axis through various mechanisms. Here's a closer look at how gut health and the microbiome can impact cortisol levels:

Microbial Metabolites and Neurotransmitters:

The microbiome produces a wide array of metabolites and neurotransmitters that can influence the stress response, including cortisol levels. For example, certain beneficial gut bacteria produce short-chain fatty acids (SCFAs), such as butyrate, which have been shown to help regulate the stress response and cortisol levels. Additionally, microbes in the gut can produce neurotransmitters, such as gamma-aminobutyric acid (GABA) and serotonin, which play a role in mood regulation and can indirectly impact cortisol levels.

Immune System Modulation:

The gut microbiome plays a crucial role in immune system regulation. Imbalances in gut microbial composition, known as dysbiosis, can trigger an inappropriate immune response, leading to chronic inflammation. Chronic inflammation, in turn, can dysregulate cortisol levels and contribute to increased stress response. By promoting a healthy balance of gut microbes, we can support proper immune system function and cortisol regulation.

Gut Permeability and Inflammation:

An unhealthy gut lining with increased permeability, known as leaky gut, can contribute to inflammation and activation of the stress response. When the gut becomes permeable, harmful substances, such as toxins and bacterial byproducts, can leak into the bloodstream, triggering an immune response and potentially leading to elevated cortisol levels. Maintaining gut health and integrity is crucial for minimizing the risk of leaky gut and its impact on cortisol regulation.

Neurotransmitter Signaling:

The gut microbiome can influence the production and signaling of neurotransmitters involved in the stress response, such as serotonin, dopamine, and GABA. Imbalances in these neurotransmitters can affect mood and stress levels, subsequently impacting cortisol production. By supporting a healthy gut microbiome, we can optimize neurotransmitter signaling and promote more balanced cortisol levels.

Managing Gut Health and Supporting Cortisol Regulation:

Maintaining a healthy gut and microbiome is crucial for supporting cortisol regulation and overall well-being. Here are some strategies to manage gut health and promote a healthier stress response:

Balanced Diet:

Adopt a balanced diet that supports a diverse and thriving gut microbiome. Include a variety of fiber-rich foods, such as fruits, vegetables, whole grains, legumes, and nuts. These foods serve as prebiotics, nourishing the beneficial bacteria in the gut. Additionally, include fermented foods, such as yogurt, kefir, sauerkraut, and kimchi, which provide probiotics that contribute to a healthy microbial balance.

Probiotic Supplementation:

Consider probiotic supplementation, especially during times of stress or antibiotic use, to support the diversity and abundance of beneficial gut bacteria. Consult with healthcare professionals for personalized recommendations based on your specific needs and health conditions.

Minimize Stress:

Stress can negatively impact gut health and the microbiome, influencing cortisol levels. Incorporate stress reduction techniques such as meditation, deep breathing exercises, yoga, or mindfulness practices into your daily routine. Regular physical activity, adequate sleep, and engaging in activities that bring you joy, and relaxation can also help manage stress and support gut health.

Minimize Antibiotic Use:

Antibiotics can disrupt the balance of gut bacteria, leading to dysbiosis. Whenever possible, minimize unnecessary antibiotic use and, if needed, work with healthcare professionals to explore alternatives or strategies to mitigate the impact on the microbiome. When antibiotics are necessary, consider probiotic supplementation during and after treatment to help restore a healthy microbial balance.

Avoid Toxins and Food Sensitivities:

Minimize exposure to environmental toxins, such as pesticides, pollutants, and chemicals, which can disrupt gut health and contribute to inflammation. Additionally, identify and avoid any food sensitivities or intolerances that may be triggering gut-related inflammation and impacting cortisol regulation.

Seek Professional Guidance:

If you have persistent gut health issues or suspect imbalances in cortisol levels, consult with healthcare professionals who specialize in gut health, such as gastroenterologists or functional medicine practitioners. They can provide guidance, conduct appropriate evaluations, and develop a personalized treatment plan that addresses both gut health and cortisol regulation.

So,

The gut and its resident microbiome play a significant role in influencing cortisol levels through the gut-brain axis. By supporting a healthy gut and a diverse microbiome through a balanced diet, stress reduction techniques, minimizing antibiotic use, avoiding toxins and food sensitivities, and seeking professional guidance, when necessary, individuals can promote a healthier stress response and cortisol regulation.

Remember, the gut-brain axis and its impact on cortisol levels are complex, and individual responses may vary. By adopting a holistic approach that encompasses lifestyle modifications, dietary choices, stress management, and personalized care, individuals can optimize their gut health and support a healthier stress response, ultimately promoting overall well-being.

Chapter 28: The Effects of Cortisol on the Thyroid Gland and Its Function

We will explore the intriguing relationship between cortisol and the thyroid gland. Cortisol, commonly known as the "stress hormone," plays a crucial role in our body's stress response and various physiological processes. The thyroid gland, on the other hand, is a butterfly-shaped gland located in the neck that produces hormones vital for metabolism, growth, and development. In this chapter, we will delve into the details of how cortisol influences the thyroid gland and its function, shedding light on the mechanisms involved and offering insights into understanding and managing the effects of cortisol on thyroid health.

Understanding the Thyroid Gland and its Function:

Before we delve into the specifics of cortisol and the thyroid gland, let's establish a foundational understanding of the thyroid. The thyroid gland produces hormones, primarily thyroxine (T4) and triiodothyronine (T3), which regulate various metabolic processes in the body. These hormones play a crucial role in maintaining energy levels, regulating body temperature, supporting growth and development, and influencing the function of many organs and tissues.

Cortisol and Thyroid Function:

Cortisol can influence thyroid function through various mechanisms. Here's a closer look at how cortisol impacts the thyroid gland:

Regulation of Thyroid Hormone Production:

Cortisol can influence the production and conversion of thyroid hormones. Cortisol can inhibit the release of thyrotropin-releasing hormone (TRH) from the hypothalamus, which is an essential factor in stimulating the release of thyroid-stimulating hormone (TSH) from the pituitary gland. Decreased TRH and TSH levels can, in turn, reduce the production and release of thyroid hormones. This mechanism is part of the body's adaptive response to stress, redirecting energy resources away from non-essential processes.

Alteration of Thyroid Hormone Conversion:

Cortisol can affect the conversion of thyroid hormones from T4 to T3. T4 is the inactive form of thyroid hormone, and it needs to be converted to T3, the active form, in order to exert its full effects on target tissues. Cortisol can inhibit the enzyme responsible for this conversion, known as 5'-deiodinase. As a result, the conversion of T4 to T3 may be impaired, leading to reduced availability of active thyroid hormone.

Impact on Thyroid Binding Proteins:

Cortisol can influence the levels and activity of thyroid-binding proteins, which transport thyroid hormones in the bloodstream. Elevated cortisol levels can increase the production of binding proteins, such as thyroid-binding globulin (TBG). When more thyroid hormones bind to these proteins, they become less available for cellular uptake and utilization, potentially leading to altered thyroid hormone function.

Immune System Modulation:

Cortisol can modulate the immune system, and imbalances in immune function can impact the thyroid gland. Conditions such as autoimmune thyroid diseases, including Hashimoto's thyroiditis and Graves' disease, involve an abnormal immune response targeting the thyroid gland. Cortisol's anti-inflammatory properties can help regulate immune function, potentially reducing inflammation and autoimmunity in the thyroid gland.

Managing Cortisol and Supporting Thyroid Health:

Maintaining a healthy balance in cortisol levels is crucial for supporting thyroid function and overall thyroid health. Here are some strategies to manage cortisol and promote a healthier thyroid:

Stress Reduction Techniques:

Engage in stress reduction techniques such as meditation, deep breathing exercises, yoga, or mindfulness practices. Chronic stress can lead to dysregulation of cortisol levels, potentially impacting thyroid function. By managing stress, cortisol levels can be regulated, supporting a healthier thyroid.

Balanced Diet:

Adopt a balanced diet that supports optimal thyroid function. Include foods rich in iodine, selenium, zinc, and vitamin D, which are important nutrients for thyroid health. Incorporate sources of healthy fats, such as omega-3 fatty acids found in fatty fish, flaxseeds, and walnuts, as they support thyroid hormone production and balance. Consult with healthcare professionals or registered dietitians for personalized dietary recommendations.

Regular Physical Activity:

Incorporate regular physical activity into your routine. Exercise has been shown to have positive effects on thyroid function by enhancing metabolism and hormone regulation. Consult with healthcare professionals for personalized exercise recommendations based on your specific needs and health conditions.

Medication and Treatment:

If you have an underlying thyroid condition, work closely with healthcare professionals, such as endocrinologists or thyroid specialists, to ensure appropriate medication and treatment. Thyroid hormone replacement therapy may be necessary if there are deficiencies or imbalances in thyroid hormone levels. Proper medication management can help optimize thyroid function alongside cortisol regulation.

Supportive Lifestyle Factors:

Maintain a healthy lifestyle that supports overall well-being. This includes getting adequate sleep, managing weight through a balanced diet and regular physical activity, and avoiding smoking and excessive ... consumption. These lifestyle factors contribute to optimal hormonal balance and overall thyroid health.

Consultation with Healthcare Professionals:

If you have concerns about your thyroid function or suspect imbalances in cortisol levels, consult with healthcare professionals who specialize in thyroid health or endocrinology. They can provide a comprehensive evaluation, diagnose underlying conditions, and develop a personalized treatment plan that addresses both thyroid function and cortisol regulation.

So,

Cortisol, the stress hormone, can influence thyroid function through its effects on thyroid hormone production, conversion, binding proteins, and immune modulation. By managing cortisol through stress reduction techniques, a balanced diet, regular physical activity, appropriate medication and treatment, supportive lifestyle factors, and seeking professional guidance, when necessary, individuals can support a healthier thyroid and optimize overall thyroid function.

Remember, the relationship between cortisol and the thyroid gland is complex, and individual responses may vary. By adopting a holistic approach that encompasses lifestyle modifications, personalized care, and ongoing monitoring, individuals can optimize their thyroid health and support a balanced interaction between cortisol and the thyroid gland.

Chapter 29: The Role of Cortisol in the Development and Progression of Autoimmune Diseases

We will explore the intriguing relationship between cortisol and autoimmune diseases. Cortisol, commonly known as the "stress hormone," plays a crucial role in our body's stress response and various physiological processes. Autoimmune diseases, on the other hand, are a group of disorders characterized by an abnormal immune response, where the immune system mistakenly attacks healthy cells and tissues. In this chapter, we will delve into the details of how cortisol influences the development and progression of autoimmune diseases, shedding light on the mechanisms involved and offering insights into understanding and managing the effects of cortisol on these complex conditions.

Understanding Autoimmune Diseases:

Before we delve into the specifics of cortisol and autoimmune diseases, let's establish a foundational understanding of these conditions. Autoimmune diseases occur when the immune system, which is designed to protect the body against foreign invaders, mistakenly targets and attacks healthy cells and tissues. There are more than 80 different types of autoimmune diseases, including rheumatoid arthritis, lupus, multiple sclerosis, type 1 diabetes, and Hashimoto's thyroiditis, among others. These diseases can affect various organs and tissues, leading to a wide range of symptoms and complications.

Cortisol and Autoimmune Diseases:

Cortisol can influence the development and progression of autoimmune diseases through various mechanisms. Here's a closer look at how cortisol impacts autoimmune diseases:

Immune System Modulation:

Cortisol has potent anti-inflammatory and immunosuppressive effects. In situations of acute stress, cortisol levels rise, temporarily suppressing the immune system's inflammatory response. This can help prevent excessive inflammation and tissue damage. However, chronic, or prolonged elevation of cortisol due to chronic stress can dysregulate the immune system, leading to imbalances and potential dysfunctions. In some cases, this dysregulation can contribute to the development or exacerbation of autoimmune diseases.

Impact on Immune Cells:

Cortisol can influence the function and activity of various immune cells involved in the development and progression of autoimmune diseases. For example, cortisol can suppress the activation and proliferation of certain T cells, which play a role in initiating and maintaining immune responses. Additionally, cortisol can modulate the production and activity of pro-inflammatory cytokines, which are molecules that promote inflammation. Imbalances in these immune cells and cytokines can contribute to autoimmune processes.

Gut Microbiome Interaction:

The gut microbiome, which consists of trillions of microorganisms in our gastrointestinal tract, plays a crucial role in immune system regulation. Imbalances in the gut microbiome, known as dysbiosis, can influence the development of autoimmune diseases. Cortisol, through its effects on the gut-brain axis, can impact the composition and diversity of the gut microbiome. Disruptions in the gut microbiome can alter immune system function and contribute to autoimmune processes.

Neuroendocrine Regulation:

The complex interplay between the nervous and endocrine systems can influence autoimmune diseases. Cortisol, as a key hormone involved in the stress response, can interact with the nervous system, and influence the release of neurotransmitters and neuropeptides that modulate immune function. Imbalances in these neuroendocrine interactions can contribute to dysregulation of the immune system and the development or progression of autoimmune diseases.

Managing Cortisol and Supporting Autoimmune Health:

Maintaining a healthy balance in cortisol levels is crucial for managing autoimmune diseases effectively. Here are some strategies to manage cortisol and promote a healthier autoimmune response:

Stress Reduction Techniques:

Engage in stress reduction techniques such as meditation, deep breathing exercises, yoga, or mindfulness practices. Chronic stress can lead to dysregulation of cortisol levels and contribute to autoimmune dysfunction. By managing stress, cortisol levels can be regulated, potentially supporting a healthier autoimmune response.

Balanced Diet:

Adopt a balanced diet that supports overall health and immune system function. Include a variety of fruits, vegetables, whole grains, lean proteins, and healthy fats. Incorporate foods rich in antioxidants and anti-inflammatory properties, such as berries, leafy greens, turmeric, ginger, and fatty fish. Consult with healthcare professionals or registered dietitians for personalized dietary recommendations based on your specific needs and health conditions.

Regular Physical Activity:

Incorporate regular physical activity into your routine. Exercise has been shown to have positive effects on immune system function and overall well-being. Consult with healthcare professionals for personalized exercise recommendations based on your specific needs and health conditions.

Adequate Sleep:

Prioritize adequate sleep to support immune system health and cortisol regulation. Aim for a consistent sleep schedule and create a sleep-friendly environment. Practice good sleep hygiene, such as avoiding electronic devices before bed, keeping the bedroom dark and quiet, and establishing a relaxing bedtime routine.

Supportive Lifestyle Factors:

Maintain a healthy lifestyle that supports overall well-being and immune system health. Avoid smoking and excessive ... consumption, as they can negatively impact immune function. Practice good hygiene and take appropriate measures to prevent infections, as infections can trigger or worsen autoimmune flares.

Consultation with Healthcare Professionals:

If you have been diagnosed with an autoimmune disease or suspect autoimmune dysfunction, work closely with healthcare professionals who specialize in autoimmune diseases, such as rheumatologists or immunologists. They can provide a comprehensive evaluation, diagnose underlying conditions, and develop a personalized treatment plan that addresses both autoimmune health and cortisol regulation.

So,

Cortisol, the stress hormone, can influence the development and progression of autoimmune diseases through its effects on the immune system, gut health, neuroendocrine regulation, and stress response. By managing cortisol through stress reduction techniques, a balanced diet, regular physical activity, adequate sleep, supportive lifestyle factors, and seeking professional guidance, when necessary, individuals can support a healthier autoimmune response and optimize their overall well-being.

Remember, autoimmune diseases are complex and multifactorial, and individual responses may vary. By adopting a holistic approach that encompasses lifestyle modifications, personalized care, and ongoing monitoring, individuals can optimize their autoimmune health and manage the effects of cortisol on these challenging conditions.

Chapter 30: The Influence of Cortisol on the Body's Response to Exercise and Physical Activity

We will explore the fascinating relationship between cortisol and the body's response to exercise and physical activity. Cortisol, commonly known as the "stress hormone," plays a crucial role in our body's stress response and various physiological processes. Exercise and physical activity, on the other hand, are essential components of a healthy lifestyle, providing numerous benefits for our physical and mental well-being. In this chapter, we will delve into the details of how cortisol influences the body's response to exercise, shedding light on the mechanisms involved and offering insights into understanding and managing the effects of cortisol on our active endeavors.

Understanding Cortisol and Exercise:

Before we delve into the specifics of cortisol and exercise, let's establish a foundational understanding of cortisol's role in the body. Cortisol is a hormone produced by the adrenal glands in response to stress. It helps regulate various physiological processes, including metabolism, immune function, blood sugar levels, and inflammation. During exercise, cortisol levels can fluctuate due to the body's stress response to physical exertion and energy demands. The effects of cortisol on exercise can vary depending on several factors, such as exercise intensity, duration, and individual characteristics.

Cortisol's Role in Exercise:

Cortisol plays several roles in the body's response to exercise. Here's a closer look at how cortisol influences exercise and physical activity:

Energy Mobilization:

During exercise, cortisol plays a role in mobilizing energy reserves. It promotes the breakdown of glycogen (stored glucose) in the liver and muscles to provide fuel for working muscles. Cortisol also stimulates the release of fatty acids from adipose tissue, which can serve as an additional energy source during prolonged exercise. This energy mobilization ensures that the body has the necessary resources to meet the increased energy demands of physical activity.

Muscle Protein Breakdown:

Cortisol can stimulate muscle protein breakdown, particularly during prolonged or intense exercise. This is a natural response to provide amino acids that can be converted into glucose to maintain blood sugar levels and support energy production. However, excessive, or prolonged cortisol elevation can contribute to muscle catabolism, which is the breakdown of muscle tissue. This is why it's important to balance exercise intensity and duration to prevent excessive cortisol release and minimize muscle breakdown.

Anti-inflammatory Effects:

While cortisol is commonly associated with stress and inflammation, it also has anti-inflammatory properties. During exercise, cortisol can help regulate the inflammatory response by reducing the production of pro-inflammatory substances. This can support tissue repair and recovery post-exercise. However, chronic, or excessive cortisol elevation due to overtraining or other factors can lead to imbalances in the inflammatory response and potentially contribute to inflammation-related issues.

Immune System Modulation:

Exercise can temporarily suppress the immune system, making individuals more susceptible to infections. Cortisol, as an immunosuppressive hormone, can further impact immune function during exercise. Moderate exercise typically leads to a temporary cortisol increase, which can have a positive effect on immune function by mobilizing immune cells. However, prolonged, or intense exercise, especially without proper recovery, can dysregulate cortisol levels and compromise immune function.

Managing Cortisol during Exercise:

Maintaining a healthy balance in cortisol levels during exercise is crucial for optimizing performance, recovery, and overall well-being. Here are some strategies to manage cortisol during exercise and physical activity:

Warm-Up and Cool-Down:

Start each exercise session with a proper warm-up and end with a cool-down. A warm-up prepares the body for physical activity, gradually increasing heart rate and body temperature. This can help minimize cortisol spikes associated with sudden exertion. Cooling down allows the body to gradually return to a resting state, facilitating recovery and minimizing cortisol elevation.

Individualized Exercise Prescription:

Design an exercise program that matches your fitness level, goals, and abilities. Gradually progress the intensity and duration of your workouts to avoid excessive cortisol release. Incorporate a mix of aerobic, strength, and flexibility exercises to promote overall fitness and minimize the risk of overtraining.

Rest and Recovery:

Allow for adequate rest and recovery between exercise sessions. This includes incorporating rest days into your exercise routine and ensuring sufficient sleep. Rest and recovery periods help balance cortisol levels, promote muscle repair, and support immune function. Listening to your body and adjusting your exercise routine accordingly is key to preventing excessive cortisol release.

Proper Nutrition:

Fuel your body with a balanced diet that supports exercise and recovery. Adequate nutrition, including a combination of carbohydrates, proteins, and healthy fats, helps maintain stable blood sugar levels and provides the necessary building blocks for muscle repair. Consult with healthcare professionals or registered dietitians for personalized dietary recommendations based on your specific needs and exercise goals.

Stress Management Techniques:

Engage in stress management techniques such as meditation, deep breathing exercises, yoga, or mindfulness practices. Chronic stress can contribute to dysregulation of cortisol levels, impacting exercise performance and recovery. By managing stress, cortisol levels can be regulated, supporting a healthier exercise response.

Hydration:

Maintain proper hydration before, during, and after exercise. Dehydration can increase cortisol release and impair exercise performance. Aim to drink sufficient fluids, especially during intense or prolonged exercise, and listen to your body's thirst cues.

So,

Cortisol, the stress hormone, plays a complex role in the body's response to exercise and physical activity. By understanding cortisol's influence on energy mobilization, muscle protein breakdown, inflammation, and immune function, individuals can optimize their exercise routine and support a healthier response to physical exertion. Remember, exercise is an important component of a healthy lifestyle, and cortisol's effects can vary based on exercise intensity, duration, and individual characteristics. By adopting a balanced approach that encompasses individualized exercise prescription, proper warm-up and cool-down, rest and recovery, proper nutrition, stress management techniques, and hydration, individuals can manage cortisol levels during exercise and promote overall well-being.

Chapter 31: The Impact of Cortisol on Fertility and Reproductive Health

We will explore the fascinating relationship between cortisol and fertility/reproductive health. Cortisol, commonly known as the "stress hormone," plays a crucial role in our body's stress response and various physiological processes. Fertility and reproductive health are vital aspects of overall well-being, and understanding the impact of cortisol on these areas is essential. In this chapter, we will delve into the details of how cortisol influences fertility and reproductive health, shedding light on the mechanisms involved and offering insights into understanding and managing the effects of cortisol on these crucial aspects of life.

Understanding Cortisol and Reproductive Health:

Before we delve into the specifics of cortisol and reproductive health, let's establish a foundational understanding of these terms. Cortisol is a hormone produced by the adrenal glands in response to stress. It helps regulate various physiological processes, including metabolism, immune function, blood pressure, and inflammation. Reproductive health refers to the state of well-being related to the reproductive system, encompassing fertility, hormonal balance, menstrual health, and overall reproductive function.

Cortisol's Influence on Fertility:

Cortisol can impact fertility through various mechanisms. Here's a closer look at how cortisol influences fertility:

Disruption of the Hypothalamic-Pituitary-Gonadal (HPG) Axis:

The hypothalamic-pituitary-gonadal (HPG) axis is a complex system involving the hypothalamus, pituitary gland, and gonads (ovaries in females and testes in males). This axis regulates the release of reproductive hormones, such as follicle-stimulating hormone (FSH) and luteinizing hormone (LH), which are essential for ovarian follicle development and ovulation in females, and testosterone production in males. Chronic stress and elevated cortisol levels can disrupt the HPG axis, leading to imbalances in reproductive hormone production and potentially affecting fertility.

Menstrual Irregularities and Anovulation:

Chronic stress and elevated cortisol levels can disrupt the normal menstrual cycle. Cortisol can inhibit the release of gonadotropin-releasing hormone (GnRH) from the hypothalamus, which is necessary for the production of FSH and LH. This disruption can result in menstrual irregularities, such as amenorrhea (absence of menstrual periods) or oligomenorrhea (infrequent or irregular menstrual periods). Additionally, anovulation, the absence of ovulation, can occur due to cortisol dysregulation, affecting fertility.

Impact on Ovarian Function:

Elevated cortisol levels can impact ovarian function and follicle development. Cortisol can interfere with the growth and maturation of ovarian follicles, which contain the eggs. This interference can lead to reduced quality and quantity of eggs, potentially affecting fertility. Additionally, cortisol dysregulation can impair the process of ovulation, further compromising fertility.

Imbalances in Reproductive Hormones:

Cortisol dysregulation can disrupt the balance of reproductive hormones, including estrogen and progesterone in females, and testosterone in males. Imbalances in these hormones can impact fertility by affecting the development and release of eggs in females, and sperm production and function in males.

Cortisol's Impact on Reproductive Health:

Apart from fertility, cortisol can impact various aspects of reproductive health. Here are some key effects:

Menstrual Disorders:

Chronic stress and elevated cortisol levels can contribute to menstrual disorders, such as irregular or absent periods, heavy or prolonged periods, or premenstrual syndrome (PMS). These menstrual disorders can be influenced by cortisol's effects on the HPG axis, ovarian function, and hormonal balance.

Sexual Dysfunction:

Elevated cortisol levels can contribute to sexual dysfunction, including decreased libido, erectile dysfunction in males, and decreased arousal and orgasmic difficulties in both males and females. Chronic stress and cortisol dysregulation can interfere with the normal physiological and psychological processes involved in sexual function.

Pregnancy Complications:

Cortisol dysregulation can increase the risk of pregnancy complications. Elevated cortisol levels can affect implantation of the fertilized egg in the uterus, increase the risk of miscarriage, and contribute to gestational diabetes and preeclampsia. Managing cortisol levels during pregnancy is crucial for ensuring optimal maternal and fetal health.

Managing Cortisol and Promoting Reproductive Health:

If you are concerned about the impact of cortisol on fertility and reproductive health, it's important to consider strategies for managing cortisol and promoting reproductive well-being. Here are some recommendations:

Stress Reduction Techniques:

Engage in stress reduction techniques such as meditation, deep breathing exercises, yoga, or mindfulness practices. By managing stress and cortisol levels, you can support reproductive health. Incorporate relaxation techniques into your daily routine and prioritize self-care activities that promote emotional well-being.

Adequate Sleep:

Prioritize good sleep hygiene practices to support cortisol regulation and reproductive health. Aim for a consistent sleep schedule, create a sleep-friendly environment, and establish a relaxing bedtime routine. Sufficient sleep is crucial for hormone balance and overall well-being.

Balanced Diet and Exercise:

Adopt a balanced diet that supports overall health and hormone regulation. Include a variety of nutrient-rich foods, such as fruits, vegetables, whole grains, lean proteins, and healthy fats. Engage in regular physical activity, as exercise can help regulate cortisol levels, improve blood circulation, and support overall reproductive health.

Supportive Lifestyle Factors:

Maintain a healthy lifestyle that supports reproductive health. Avoid excessive ... consumption, smoking, and illicit drug use, as they can negatively impact fertility and reproductive function. Prioritize open communication with your healthcare provider and discuss any concerns or questions related to reproductive health.

Seeking Professional Help:

If you are experiencing difficulties with fertility or have concerns about cortisol's impact on reproductive health, seek professional help. Healthcare professionals, such as reproductive endocrinologists, gynecologists, or fertility specialists, can provide a comprehensive evaluation, diagnose underlying conditions, and develop a personalized treatment plan that addresses both cortisol regulation and reproductive health.

So,

Cortisol, the stress hormone, can impact fertility and reproductive health through its effects on the HPG axis, ovarian function, hormonal balance, and various physiological processes. By understanding the relationship between cortisol and reproductive health, individuals can make informed decisions about managing stress, optimizing hormone balance, and seeking professional guidance when necessary.

Remember, fertility and reproductive health are influenced by multiple factors, and individual responses may vary. By adopting a holistic approach that encompasses stress reduction techniques, adequate sleep, balanced diet and exercise, supportive lifestyle factors, and professional guidance, individuals can manage cortisol levels and promote reproductive well-being.

Chapter 32: The Impact of Cortisol on the Body's Response to Temperature Regulation

We will explore the intriguing relationship between cortisol and the body's response to temperature regulation. Cortisol, commonly known as the "stress hormone," plays a crucial role in our body's stress response and various physiological processes. Temperature regulation is essential for maintaining homeostasis and ensuring the body functions optimally. In this chapter, we will delve into the details of how cortisol influences the body's response to temperature changes, shedding light on the mechanisms involved and offering insights into understanding and managing the effects of cortisol on temperature regulation.

Understanding Cortisol and Temperature Regulation:

Before we delve into the specifics of cortisol and temperature regulation, let's establish a foundational understanding of these terms. Cortisol is a hormone produced by the adrenal glands in response to stress. It helps regulate various physiological processes, including metabolism, immune function, blood pressure, and inflammation. Temperature regulation, also known as thermoregulation, refers to the body's ability to maintain a stable internal temperature within a narrow range despite external temperature changes.

Cortisol's Influence on Temperature Regulation:

Cortisol can impact the body's response to temperature regulation through various mechanisms. Here's a closer look at how cortisol influences temperature regulation:

Metabolic Effects:

Cortisol plays a role in regulating metabolism, which can indirectly impact temperature regulation. Cortisol stimulates gluconeogenesis, the production of glucose from non-carbohydrate sources, which helps provide energy during stressful situations. This metabolic process generates heat as a byproduct, contributing to an increase in body temperature. Additionally, cortisol can influence metabolic rate, affecting how the body generates and dissipates heat.

Inflammatory Response:

Cortisol has anti-inflammatory properties that can modulate the body's immune response to inflammation. Inflammation can occur as a result of tissue damage or infection, and it can lead to an increase in body temperature. Cortisol helps suppress the inflammatory response, which can help regulate body temperature during inflammatory processes.

Sympathetic Nervous System Activation:

Cortisol interacts with the sympathetic nervous system, which is responsible for the body's fight-or-flight response. During periods of stress, cortisol can activate the sympathetic nervous system, leading to various physiological responses, including an increase in heart rate, blood pressure, and body temperature. This response is part of the body's adaptive mechanism to prepare for physical exertion or escape from perceived threats.

Stress-Induced Hyperthermia:

Chronic or excessive cortisol elevation due to prolonged stress can lead to stress-induced hyperthermia. Stress activates the hypothalamic-pituitary-adrenal (HPA) axis, leading to cortisol release. This stress response can result in elevated body temperature, as the body prepares for potential danger or physical exertion. Prolonged stress and elevated cortisol levels can dysregulate temperature regulation, leading to difficulties in maintaining a stable body temperature.

Effects of Cortisol on Temperature Regulation:

The influence of cortisol on temperature regulation can have several effects on the body. Here are some key effects:

Hyperthermia:

Elevated cortisol levels can contribute to hyperthermia, which is an abnormally high body temperature. This can occur as a result of prolonged stress, chronic inflammation, or metabolic disturbances. Hyperthermia can have various health consequences and may require medical intervention to regulate body temperature.

Night Sweats:

Cortisol dysregulation can lead to night sweats, which are episodes of excessive sweating during sleep. Night sweats can disrupt sleep and contribute to discomfort. They are often associated with hormonal imbalances, including cortisol dysregulation, although other factors can also contribute.

Altered Heat Perception:

Cortisol dysregulation can impact the body's perception of temperature. Individuals may experience altered sensitivity to hot or cold temperatures, feeling excessively hot or cold compared to their surroundings. This can affect their comfort and ability to adapt to different environmental temperatures.

Managing Cortisol and Supporting Temperature Regulation:

Maintaining a healthy balance in cortisol levels is crucial for supporting temperature regulation. Here are some strategies to manage cortisol and promote optimal temperature regulation:

Stress Management:

Engage in stress reduction techniques such as meditation, deep breathing exercises, yoga, or mindfulness practices. Chronic stress can contribute to cortisol dysregulation, which can impact temperature regulation. By managing stress, cortisol levels can be regulated, potentially supporting more balanced temperature responses.

Adequate Hydration:

Proper hydration is important for temperature regulation. Drink sufficient fluids, especially water, to maintain adequate hydration levels. Dehydration can hinder the body's ability to regulate body temperature effectively.

Dress Appropriately:

Wear clothing appropriate for the environmental temperature. Layer clothing to adjust to changing temperatures and allow for easy regulation of body heat. Choose fabrics that promote breathability and moisture-wicking properties to support temperature regulation.

Environmental Modifications:

Make environmental modifications to support temperature regulation. Use fans, air conditioning, or heating systems to create a comfortable environment. Consider using blankets or adjusting room temperature during sleep to support optimal sleep temperature.

Balanced Lifestyle:

Maintain a balanced lifestyle that supports overall well-being. Practice good sleep hygiene, engage in regular physical activity, eat a balanced diet, and manage stress through healthy coping mechanisms. These lifestyle factors can help support optimal cortisol regulation and temperature regulation.

Consultation with Healthcare Professionals:

If you experience chronic difficulties with temperature regulation or suspect cortisol dysregulation, consult with healthcare professionals. They can provide a comprehensive evaluation, diagnose underlying conditions, and develop a personalized treatment plan that addresses both cortisol regulation and temperature regulation.

So,

Cortisol, the stress hormone, can influence the body's response to temperature regulation through its effects on metabolism, inflammatory response, sympathetic nervous system activation, and stress-induced hyperthermia. By understanding the relationship between cortisol and temperature regulation, individuals can make informed decisions about managing stress, supporting temperature balance, and seeking professional guidance when necessary.

Remember, temperature regulation is a complex process influenced by various factors, and individual responses may vary. By adopting a holistic approach that encompasses stress management techniques, adequate hydration, appropriate clothing choices, environmental modifications, balanced lifestyle habits, and consultation with healthcare professionals, individuals can manage cortisol levels and support optimal temperature regulation.

Chapter 33: The Role of Cortisol in Mood Disorders: Depression and Bipolar Disorder

We will explore the intriguing relationship between cortisol and mood disorders, specifically depression and bipolar disorder. Cortisol, commonly known as the "stress hormone," plays a crucial role in our body's stress response and various physiological processes. Mood disorders, such as depression and bipolar disorder, are complex mental health conditions that can significantly impact an individual's emotional well-being. In this chapter, we will delve into the details of how cortisol influences these mood disorders, shedding light on the mechanisms involved and offering insights into understanding and managing the effects of cortisol on depression and bipolar disorder.

Understanding Cortisol and Mood Disorders:

Before we delve into the specifics of cortisol and mood disorders, let's establish a foundational understanding of these terms. Cortisol is a hormone produced by the adrenal glands in response to stress. It helps regulate various physiological processes, including metabolism, immune function, blood pressure, and inflammation. Mood disorders encompass a range of mental health conditions characterized by persistent disturbances in mood, affecting emotions, thoughts, and behavior.

Cortisol's Influence on Depression:

Depression is a mood disorder characterized by persistent feelings of sadness, hopelessness, and a loss of interest in activities. Cortisol can impact depression through various mechanisms. Here's a closer look at how cortisol influences depression:

Dysregulation of the Hypothalamic-Pituitary-Adrenal (HPA) Axis:

The HPA axis is a complex system involving the hypothalamus, pituitary gland, and adrenal glands, which regulates cortisol production and release. In individuals with depression, the HPA axis may be dysregulated, leading to abnormal cortisol levels. Some individuals with depression may have elevated cortisol levels, while others may exhibit blunted cortisol responses to stress.

Impact on Neurotransmitters:

Cortisol can influence neurotransmitter levels, particularly serotonin, norepinephrine, and dopamine, which play crucial roles in mood regulation. Cortisol can affect the synthesis, release, and reuptake of these neurotransmitters, potentially contributing to the development or exacerbation of depressive symptoms.

Hippocampal Volume Reduction:

Prolonged exposure to elevated cortisol levels may lead to structural changes in the brain, particularly in the hippocampus, a region involved in memory and emotion regulation. In depression, individuals may exhibit reduced hippocampal volume, potentially related to the effects of cortisol on this brain structure. The hippocampus is also involved in the regulation of the HPA axis, creating a complex interplay between cortisol, mood, and brain structures.

Disrupted Circadian Rhythm:

Cortisol follows a diurnal rhythm, with higher levels in the morning and lower levels in the evening. Individuals with depression may exhibit disruptions in their cortisol diurnal rhythm, with elevated evening cortisol levels or blunted cortisol awakening response. These disruptions can impact sleep patterns, energy levels, and mood regulation.

Cortisol's Influence on Bipolar Disorder:

Bipolar disorder is a mood disorder characterized by alternating periods of depression and mania or hypomania. Cortisol can influence bipolar disorder through various mechanisms. Here's a closer look at how cortisol influences bipolar disorder:

Cortisol Dysregulation During Mood Episodes:

During manic or depressive episodes in bipolar disorder, cortisol levels can be dysregulated. During manic episodes, individuals may exhibit elevated cortisol levels, contributing to increased energy, agitation, and sleep disturbances. During depressive episodes, cortisol dysregulation may manifest as blunted cortisol responses to stress, which can impact mood, energy levels, and cognitive function.

Impact on Stress Sensitivity:

Cortisol dysregulation in bipolar disorder can contribute to increased stress sensitivity. Individuals with bipolar disorder may exhibit heightened cortisol responses to stress, making them more vulnerable to the negative impact of stressors on mood stability. Chronic or prolonged stress can further dysregulate cortisol levels and exacerbate bipolar symptoms.

Interactions with Mood-Stabilizing Medications:

Some medications commonly used to manage bipolar disorder, such as lithium and anticonvulsants, can influence cortisol levels. These medications may modulate cortisol production and release, helping to stabilize mood and prevent episodes of mania or depression. The complex interplay between cortisol and mood-stabilizing medications is an active area of research.

Managing Cortisol and Supporting Mood Disorders:

If you are concerned about the impact of cortisol on mood disorders, such as depression or bipolar disorder, it's important to consider strategies for managing cortisol and supporting emotional well-being. Here are some recommendations:

Medication Management:

For individuals with diagnosed mood disorders, work closely with healthcare professionals to develop an individualized medication regimen. Mood-stabilizing medications, antidepressants, or other prescribed treatments can help manage symptoms and regulate cortisol levels.

Psychotherapy:

Engage in psychotherapy, such as cognitive-behavioral therapy (CBT), which can help individuals with mood disorders develop coping strategies, manage stress, and modify negative thought patterns. Psychotherapy can also contribute to cortisol regulation by addressing underlying psychological factors.

Stress Reduction Techniques:

Incorporate stress reduction techniques into daily life. Engage in activities such as meditation, mindfulness, deep breathing exercises, yoga, or relaxation techniques. These practices can help manage cortisol levels, reduce stress, and promote emotional well-being.

Regular Sleep Patterns:

Prioritize regular sleep patterns to support cortisol regulation and stabilize mood. Establish a consistent sleep schedule, create a sleep-friendly environment, and practice good sleep hygiene. Sufficient and quality sleep can positively impact mood, energy levels, and cortisol regulation.

Physical Activity:

Engage in regular physical activity, as exercise has been shown to improve mood and reduce stress. Physical activity can help regulate cortisol levels, promote the release of endorphins (feel-good hormones), and contribute to overall well-being. Find activities that you enjoy and make them a part of your routine.

Social Support:

Build a strong support network of friends, family, or support groups. Having a support system can provide emotional support, reduce feelings of isolation, and help manage stress. Social connections can positively influence cortisol regulation and contribute to overall mental well-being.

Healthy Lifestyle:

Maintain a healthy lifestyle that supports emotional well-being. Eat a balanced diet, stay hydrated, limit ... and substance use, and avoid excessive caffeine intake. These lifestyle choices can contribute to overall health and support cortisol regulation.

Self-Care:

Prioritize self-care activities that promote relaxation, joy, and self-compassion. Engage in hobbies, engage in activities that bring you pleasure and relaxation, and practice self-care rituals. Taking time for yourself can help reduce stress, support cortisol regulation, and enhance emotional well-being.

Ongoing Professional Support:

Continue to work closely with healthcare professionals specializing in mood disorders. Regular check-ins and ongoing professional support can help monitor cortisol levels, assess treatment effectiveness, and make necessary adjustments to medications or therapeutic interventions.

So,

Cortisol, the stress hormone, can play a significant role in mood disorders such as depression and bipolar disorder. By understanding the relationship between cortisol and these mood disorders, individuals can make informed decisions about managing stress, seeking appropriate treatments, and adopting strategies to support emotional well-being.

It's important to remember that mood disorders are complex and multifaceted, involving a combination of genetic, environmental, and neurobiological factors. Cortisol is just one piece of the puzzle. By working collaboratively with healthcare professionals, implementing stress reduction techniques, maintaining a healthy lifestyle, and prioritizing self-care, individuals can manage cortisol levels and support their journey towards emotional well-being.

Chapter 34: The Influence of Certain Types of Cancer on Cortisol Levels

We will explore the intriguing relationship between certain types of cancer and cortisol levels. Cortisol, commonly known as the "stress hormone," plays a crucial role in our body's stress response and various physiological processes. Cancer is a complex disease characterized by the uncontrolled growth of abnormal cells. In this chapter, we will delve into the details of how certain types of cancer can influence cortisol levels, shedding light on the mechanisms involved and offering insights into understanding and managing the effects of cancer on cortisol regulation.

Understanding Cortisol and Cancer:

Before we delve into the specifics of cortisol and cancer, let's establish a foundational understanding of these terms. Cortisol is a hormone produced by the adrenal glands in response to stress. It helps regulate various physiological processes, including metabolism, immune function, blood pressure, and inflammation. Cancer refers to a group of diseases characterized by the uncontrollable growth and spread of abnormal cells, potentially affecting various parts of the body.

Cortisol's Influence in Cancer:

Cortisol levels can be influenced by certain types of cancer, and this can occur through various mechanisms. Here's a closer look at how cancer can influence cortisol levels:

Adrenal Gland Tumors:

Certain types of tumors can develop in the adrenal glands, which are responsible for producing cortisol. Adrenal tumors, such as adrenal cortical carcinoma or adrenal adenoma, can lead to excessive cortisol production, a condition known as Cushing's syndrome. Elevated cortisol levels can contribute to various symptoms and complications, including weight gain, high blood pressure, muscle weakness, and mood changes.

Paraneoplastic Syndromes:

Paraneoplastic syndromes are a group of disorders that occur due to the production of hormone-like substances by cancer cells, often unrelated to the primary tumor site. In some cases, cancer cells can produce substances that mimic the action of cortisol or stimulate cortisol release. This can result in elevated cortisol levels and the manifestation of Cushing's syndrome-like symptoms, even in the absence of primary adrenal gland involvement.

Stress and Psychological Impact:

A cancer diagnosis and treatment can induce significant psychological and emotional stress. This stress can lead to the activation of the hypothalamic-pituitary-adrenal (HPA) axis, resulting in increased cortisol production. The psychological burden of cancer, including fear, anxiety, and depression, can contribute to cortisol dysregulation.

Inflammatory Response:

Cancer can trigger an inflammatory response in the body. Inflammation is closely interconnected with cortisol regulation, as cortisol possesses anti-inflammatory properties. In some cases, the body may produce higher levels of cortisol to combat inflammation associated with cancer. This can result in elevated cortisol levels as part of the body's immune response.

Effects of Cortisol on Cancer Progression and Symptoms:

The impact of cortisol on cancer progression and symptoms can vary depending on the specific context. Here are some key effects:

Immune Suppression:

Elevated cortisol levels can suppress the immune system, impairing the body's ability to mount an effective defense against cancer cells. This immune suppression can potentially contribute to cancer progression and compromise the effectiveness of cancer treatments.

Muscle Wasting and Weight Loss:

Excessive cortisol production can lead to muscle wasting and weight loss. In certain types of cancer, elevated cortisol levels can contribute to cachexia, a condition characterized by severe weight loss and muscle wasting. Cachexia can significantly impact a patient's quality of life and treatment outcomes.

Impact on Bone Health:

Cortisol dysregulation, particularly in cases of prolonged elevation, can contribute to bone loss and increase the risk of osteoporosis. Cancer-related hypercortisolism or prolonged exposure to high cortisol levels can have detrimental effects on bone health, potentially leading to fractures and other complications.

Psychological Impact:

Cortisol dysregulation can contribute to psychological symptoms, such as anxiety and depression, which are common in individuals diagnosed with cancer. Elevated cortisol levels can exacerbate the emotional burden of cancer and impact overall well-being.

Managing Cortisol and Supporting Cancer Treatment:

If you are concerned about the impact of cortisol on cancer or its treatment, it's important to consider strategies for managing cortisol levels and supporting the overall management of the disease. Here are some recommendations:

Medical Evaluation and Treatment:

If you suspect cortisol dysregulation due to cancer or its treatment, consult with healthcare professionals specializing in oncology. They can conduct a thorough medical evaluation, including hormone tests, and develop an individualized treatment plan to address cortisol-related concerns.

Cancer Treatment Planning:

Work closely with oncologists and healthcare professionals to develop a comprehensive cancer treatment plan. This may include surgery, chemotherapy, radiation therapy, or targeted therapies, depending on the type and stage of cancer. The primary focus should be on cancer management and control, which may indirectly impact cortisol levels.

Stress Management:

Engage in stress reduction techniques such as meditation, deep breathing exercises, yoga, or mindfulness practices. Chronic stress can contribute to cortisol dysregulation. By managing stress, cortisol levels can be regulated, potentially supporting overall well-being during cancer treatment.

Supportive Care:

Incorporate supportive care interventions into your cancer treatment plan. This may include psychological support, counseling, or participation in support groups. Addressing the psychological impact of cancer and managing emotional well-being can help reduce stress and support cortisol regulation.

Healthy Lifestyle:

Maintain a healthy lifestyle that supports overall well-being. Focus on eating a balanced diet, engaging in regular physical activity, getting adequate rest, and staying hydrated. These lifestyle factors can contribute to overall health, improve treatment outcomes, and indirectly impact cortisol regulation.

Social Support:

Build a strong support network of friends, family, or support groups. Having a support system can provide emotional support, reduce feelings of isolation, and help manage stress. Social connections can positively influence cortisol regulation and contribute to overall well-being during cancer treatment.

Ongoing Communication with Healthcare Professionals:

Maintain open and ongoing communication with healthcare professionals involved in your cancer care. Discuss any concerns or questions related to cortisol levels, treatment side effects, or psychological well-being. Regular check-ins and open dialogue can help ensure that appropriate measures are taken to address cortisol-related issues.

So,

Certain types of cancer can influence cortisol levels through various mechanisms, such as adrenal tumors, paraneoplastic syndromes, stress-induced activation of the HPA axis, and the inflammatory response. The impact of cortisol on cancer progression and symptoms can be diverse, affecting immune function, muscle wasting, bone health, and psychological well-being.

If you suspect cortisol dysregulation or have concerns about its impact on cancer, it's important to work closely with healthcare professionals specializing in oncology. They can provide a thorough evaluation, develop an individualized treatment plan, and offer support to manage cortisol-related concerns alongside cancer treatment.

Remember, managing cortisol levels in the context of cancer is a complex task, and individual responses may vary. By adopting a comprehensive approach that encompasses medical evaluation and treatment, stress management techniques, supportive care, healthy lifestyle practices, social support, and ongoing communication with healthcare professionals, individuals can navigate the intricacies of cortisol and cancer while focusing on overall well-being and cancer management.

Chapter 35: The Fascinating Connection Between Cortisol and the Gut-Brain Axis

We will explore the intriguing relationship between cortisol and the gut-brain axis. Cortisol, commonly known as the "stress hormone," plays a crucial role in our body's stress response and various physiological processes. The gut-brain axis refers to the bidirectional communication system between the gastrointestinal tract and the brain. In this chapter, we will delve into the details of how cortisol influences the gut-brain axis, shedding light on the mechanisms involved and offering insights into understanding and managing the effects of cortisol on gut health and mental well-being.

Understanding Cortisol and the Gut-Brain Axis:

Before we delve into the specifics of cortisol and the gut-brain axis, let's establish a foundational understanding of these terms. Cortisol is a hormone produced by the adrenal glands in response to stress. It helps regulate various physiological processes, including metabolism, immune function, blood pressure, and inflammation. The gut-brain axis refers to the complex interplay between the gut, which includes the gastrointestinal tract and its resident microbes, and the brain, encompassing neural, hormonal, and immune pathways that facilitate communication between these two systems.

Cortisol's Influence on the Gut-Brain Axis:

Cortisol can influence the gut-brain axis through various mechanisms. Here's a closer look at how cortisol influences this intricate connection:

Stress Response and HPA Axis Activation:

When we experience stress, cortisol is released as part of the body's stress response. This release of cortisol is orchestrated by the hypothalamic-pituitary-adrenal (HPA) axis, a complex network involving the hypothalamus, pituitary gland, and adrenal glands. Stress-induced activation of the HPA axis can impact the gut-brain axis, as cortisol influences both gut function and brain activity.

Gut Barrier Integrity:

Cortisol can affect the integrity of the gut barrier, which consists of a protective layer of cells that line the gastrointestinal tract.

Chronic or excessive cortisol exposure can compromise the gut barrier, leading to increased permeability, often referred to as "leaky gut." This increased permeability allows substances, such as bacteria, toxins, and undigested food particles, to pass through the gut lining and enter the bloodstream, triggering an immune response and potentially impacting brain function.

Gut Microbiota:

The gut microbiota, the vast community of microorganisms residing in the gastrointestinal tract, plays a crucial role in gut-brain communication. Cortisol can influence the composition and diversity of the gut microbiota. Elevated cortisol levels, particularly during periods of chronic stress, can disrupt the balance of beneficial and harmful bacteria in the gut, potentially impacting the overall health of the gut microbiota and subsequently affecting the gut-brain axis.

Inflammation and Immune Response:

Cortisol possesses anti-inflammatory properties and can modulate immune responses. In the gut, cortisol can impact inflammation and immune activation. Chronic or excessive cortisol levels can contribute to low-grade inflammation in the gut, which may interfere with normal gut function and disrupt the delicate balance of the gut-brain axis. Inflammation can influence brain function and mood, potentially contributing to mental health disorders.

Effects of Cortisol on Gut Health and Mental Well-being:

The impact of cortisol on the gut-brain axis can have several effects on gut health and mental well-being. Here are some key effects:

Gastrointestinal Symptoms:

Elevated cortisol levels can contribute to gastrointestinal symptoms, including abdominal pain, bloating, diarrhea, and constipation. These symptoms may arise due to cortisol's impact on gut motility, gut barrier integrity, and gut microbial balance.

Mental Health Disorders:

Dysregulation of the gut-brain axis, influenced by cortisol, has been linked to mental health disorders such as anxiety, depression, and even neurodevelopmental conditions like autism spectrum disorder. Cortisol dysregulation can impact neurotransmitter balance, immune function, and inflammation, all of which play crucial roles in mental well-being.

Altered Eating Patterns:

Cortisol can influence eating behaviors and appetite. Elevated cortisol levels can contribute to cravings for high-calorie and carbohydrate-rich foods, potentially leading to weight gain and disrupted eating patterns. These changes in eating behaviors can further impact gut health and mental well-being.

Systemic Inflammation:

Increased cortisol levels and gut inflammation can contribute to systemic inflammation, which has been associated with various chronic conditions, including cardiovascular disease, diabetes, and autoimmune disorders. Systemic inflammation can affect both gut health and mental well-being.

Managing Cortisol and Supporting the Gut-Brain Axis:

To support a healthy gut-brain axis and manage cortisol levels, it's important to consider strategies that promote gut health and overall well-being. Here are some recommendations:

Stress Management:

Engage in stress reduction techniques such as meditation, deep breathing exercises, yoga, or mindfulness practices. Chronic stress can contribute to cortisol dysregulation, impacting the gut-brain axis. By managing stress, cortisol levels can be regulated, potentially supporting a healthy gut-brain connection.

Balanced Diet:

Adopt balanced and varied diet rich in whole foods, including fruits, vegetables, whole grains, lean proteins, and healthy fats. A diverse diet can support a healthy gut microbiota, which is crucial for gut-brain communication. Include prebiotic and probiotic-rich foods to nourish and maintain a healthy gut microbial community.

Regular Physical Activity:

Engage in regular physical activity, as exercise has been shown to positively influence gut health and mental well-being. Exercise can help regulate cortisol levels, improve gut motility, and enhance the diversity of the gut microbiota. Find activities that you enjoy and make them a part of your routine.

Adequate Sleep:

Prioritize good sleep hygiene and aim for sufficient and restorative sleep. Sleep deprivation can contribute to increased cortisol levels and disrupt the delicate balance of the gut-brain axis. Establish a consistent sleep schedule, create a sleep-friendly environment, and practice relaxation techniques to support quality sleep.

Mindful Eating:

Practice mindful eating by paying attention to your body's hunger and fullness cues, eating slowly, and savoring each bite. Mindful eating can promote healthy eating patterns, improve digestion, and support the gut-brain axis.

Social Connection:

Nurture social connections and maintain a supportive network of friends, family, or support groups. Positive social interactions and social support can positively impact mental well-being and indirectly influence cortisol regulation and gut health.

Consultation with Healthcare Professionals:

If you experience persistent gastrointestinal symptoms or mental health concerns, consult with healthcare professionals specializing in gastroenterology or mental health. They can provide a comprehensive evaluation, diagnose underlying conditions, and develop a personalized treatment plan that addresses cortisol regulation and supports the gut-brain axis.

So,

Cortisol, as a key player in the stress response, can significantly influence the gut-brain axis, impacting gut health and mental well-being. By understanding the intricate connection between cortisol and the gut-brain axis, individuals can make informed decisions about managing stress, adopting a healthy lifestyle, and seeking professional guidance when necessary.

Remember, the gut-brain axis is a complex system influenced by various factors, and individual responses may vary. By adopting a holistic approach that encompasses stress management techniques, a balanced diet, regular physical activity, adequate sleep, mindful eating, social connection, and ongoing communication with healthcare professionals, individuals can support a healthy gut-brain axis and promote optimal gut health and mental wellbeing. Nurturing this connection can have profound effects on overall well-being and pave the way for a healthier and more harmonious relationship between the gut and the brain.

Chapter 36: The Influence of Cortisol on Allergies and Allergic Reactions

We will explore the fascinating relationship between cortisol and allergies. Cortisol, commonly known as the "stress hormone," plays a crucial role in our body's stress response and various physiological processes. Allergies are immune responses triggered by exposure to certain substances, known as allergens, that are typically harmless to most individuals. In this chapter, we will delve into the details of how cortisol influences the body's response to allergies and allergic reactions, shedding light on the mechanisms involved and offering insights into understanding and managing the effects of cortisol on allergic conditions.

Understanding Cortisol and Allergic Reactions:

Before we delve into the specifics of cortisol and allergies, let's establish a foundational understanding of these terms. Cortisol is a hormone produced by the adrenal glands in response to stress. It helps regulate various physiological processes, including metabolism, immune function, blood pressure, and inflammation. Allergic reactions occur when the immune system overreacts to typically harmless substances, such as pollen, pet dander, or certain foods, resulting in symptoms ranging from mild discomfort to severe reactions.

Cortisol's Influence on Allergic Reactions:

Cortisol can influence the body's response to allergic reactions through various mechanisms. Here's a closer look at how cortisol influences this intricate connection:

Anti-inflammatory Effects:

Cortisol possesses potent anti-inflammatory properties. When the immune system recognizes an allergen as a threat, it releases chemicals, including histamines, that cause inflammation and trigger allergic symptoms. Cortisol helps counteract this inflammation by suppressing the immune response and reducing the release of inflammatory mediators. It can help alleviate the symptoms associated with allergic reactions, such as redness, swelling, itching, and discomfort.

Immune Modulation:

Cortisol plays a role in modulating immune responses. In the case of allergies, cortisol can help regulate the immune system's reaction to allergens. It can help prevent excessive immune activation and the production of an exaggerated response to harmless substances. This immune modulation can reduce the severity of allergic reactions and promote a more balanced immune response.

Stress and Allergic Reactions:

Stress can influence allergic reactions, and cortisol plays a significant role in the stress response. When the body is under stress, cortisol levels rise. Stress-induced cortisol release can impact the immune system and alter immune responses, potentially exacerbating allergic reactions. Individuals with chronic stress may experience more frequent or severe allergic symptoms due to the impact of cortisol on immune function.

Allergic Sensitization:

Cortisol may also play a role in the process of allergic sensitization, which refers to the initial development of an allergic response to a specific allergen. During sensitization, the immune system becomes hypersensitive to an allergen, leading to subsequent allergic reactions upon exposure. Cortisol's anti-inflammatory properties may help modulate the immune system's response during the sensitization process, potentially influencing the development of allergies.

Effects of Cortisol on Allergic Conditions:

The impact of cortisol on allergic conditions can have several effects on the body's response to allergens and allergic reactions. Here are some key effects:

Symptom Relief:

Cortisol's anti-inflammatory effects can provide relief from allergic symptoms, such as itching, sneezing, nasal congestion, skin rashes, and respiratory difficulties. Corticosteroid medications that mimic the action of cortisol, such as nasal sprays, inhalers, or topical creams, are commonly prescribed to reduce inflammation and alleviate allergic symptoms.

Modulation of Allergic Asthma:

Allergic asthma is a type of asthma triggered by exposure to allergens. Cortisol plays a crucial role in the management of allergic asthma by reducing airway inflammation and relaxing the smooth muscles in the airways. Inhaled corticosteroids, which deliver cortisol-like medications directly to the lungs, are commonly prescribed to control allergic asthma and prevent asthma attacks.

Impact on Anaphylaxis:

Anaphylaxis is a severe and potentially life-threatening allergic reaction that can occur rapidly after exposure to an allergen. Cortisol's anti-inflammatory and immune modulatory effects may help dampen the severity of anaphylactic reactions. However, in cases of severe allergic reactions, immediate medical attention, and the administration of epinephrine (adrenaline) are critical, as cortisol alone may not be sufficient to manage the life-threatening symptoms.

Allergy Management:

Cortisol, through its influence on immune responses, can play a role in allergy management. By modulating the immune system's response to allergens, cortisol can help reduce the frequency and intensity of allergic reactions. This may involve implementing avoidance strategies for known allergens, using medications as prescribed by healthcare professionals, and managing stress levels to support overall immune balance.

Managing Cortisol and Supporting Allergy Management:

To manage cortisol levels and support allergy management, it's important to consider strategies that promote overall well-being and immune balance. Here are some recommendations:

Allergen Avoidance:

Identify and avoid exposure to allergens that trigger allergic reactions. This may involve making changes to your environment, such as using dust mite covers for bedding, keeping windows closed during high pollen seasons, or avoiding certain foods or ingredients known to cause allergies. Minimizing exposure to allergens can help reduce the frequency and severity of allergic reactions.

Medication Management:

Work closely with healthcare professionals, such as allergists or immunologists, to develop an individualized medication plan. This may include antihistamines, corticosteroids, or other prescribed medications to manage allergic symptoms. Adhering to the prescribed medication regimen can help control inflammation and alleviate allergic reactions.

Stress Reduction:

Engage in stress reduction techniques such as meditation, deep breathing exercises, yoga, or mindfulness practices. Chronic stress can impact cortisol levels and potentially exacerbate allergic reactions. By managing stress, cortisol levels can be regulated, promoting a more balanced immune response, and potentially reducing the severity of allergic symptoms.

Supportive Care:

Incorporate supportive care interventions into your allergy management plan. This may include using saline nasal rinses to alleviate nasal congestion, applying soothing creams or lotions to relieve skin irritation, or using non-medicated eye drops for allergic conjunctivitis. These supportive measures can complement medication management and provide additional relief from allergic symptoms.

Regular Communication with Healthcare Professionals:

Maintain open and ongoing communication with healthcare professionals specializing in allergies. Regular check-ins can help monitor symptoms, assess treatment effectiveness, and make necessary adjustments to medication or management strategies. Healthcare professionals can provide guidance and support tailored to your specific allergic conditions.

So,

Cortisol, with its anti-inflammatory and immune modulatory effects, plays a significant role in the body's response to allergies and allergic reactions. By understanding the influence of cortisol on allergic conditions, individuals can make informed decisions about managing stress, avoiding allergens, using appropriate medications, and seeking professional guidance when necessary.

It's important to remember that allergies are complex and individual responses may vary. Allergy management involves a comprehensive approach that encompasses allergen avoidance, medication management, stress reduction, supportive care, and ongoing communication with healthcare professionals. By adopting these strategies, individuals can navigate the intricacies of cortisol and allergies while focusing on their overall well-being and quality of life.

Chapter 37: The Intriguing Link Between Cortisol and Neurodegenerative Diseases

We will explore the fascinating relationship between cortisol and neurodegenerative diseases. Cortisol, commonly known as the "stress hormone," plays a crucial role in our body's stress response and various physiological processes. Neurodegenerative diseases are a group of disorders characterized by the progressive loss of neurons and cognitive decline. In this chapter, we will delve into the details of how cortisol influences the development and progression of neurodegenerative diseases, shedding light on the mechanisms involved and offering insights into understanding and managing the effects of cortisol on these conditions.

Understanding Cortisol and Neurodegenerative Diseases:

Before we delve into the specifics of cortisol and neurodegenerative diseases, let's establish a foundational understanding of these terms. Cortisol is a hormone produced by the adrenal glands in response to stress. It helps regulate various physiological processes, including metabolism, immune function, blood pressure, and inflammation. Neurodegenerative diseases encompass a range of conditions, such as Alzheimer's disease, Parkinson's disease, Huntington's disease, and amyotrophic lateral sclerosis (ALS), characterized by the progressive loss of neurons in specific regions of the brain.

Cortisol's Influence on Neurodegenerative Diseases:

Cortisol can influence the development and progression of neurodegenerative diseases through various mechanisms. Here's a closer look at how cortisol influences this intricate connection:

Chronic Stress and Cortisol Dysregulation:

Chronic stress can contribute to cortisol dysregulation, leading to prolonged elevation of cortisol levels in the body. Elevated cortisol levels, particularly over an extended period, can have detrimental effects on the brain. Chronic stress and cortisol dysregulation have been associated with increased susceptibility to neurodegenerative diseases and accelerated cognitive decline.

Impact on Hippocampus:

The hippocampus is a brain region crucial for memory and learning. Cortisol receptors are abundantly present in the hippocampus, and elevated cortisol levels can impact the structure and function of this region. Prolonged exposure to high cortisol levels can lead to hippocampal atrophy and impaired memory function, which are common features of neurodegenerative diseases like Alzheimer's disease.

Inflammation and Oxidative Stress:

Cortisol can modulate the body's inflammatory and oxidative stress responses. While cortisol possesses anti-inflammatory properties, prolonged elevation of cortisol levels can result in an imbalance in the inflammatory response, leading to chronic low-grade inflammation. This chronic inflammation and oxidative stress can contribute to neuronal damage and accelerate the progression of neurodegenerative diseases.

Glucocorticoid Receptor Dysfunction:

Glucocorticoid receptors, which bind cortisol, are present throughout the brain. Dysregulation of these receptors can occur in neurodegenerative diseases, affecting the brain's response to cortisol. In certain cases, the sensitivity of these receptors may be altered, leading to impaired cortisol signaling and disruption of normal cellular processes.

Effects of Cortisol on Neurodegenerative Diseases:

The impact of cortisol on neurodegenerative diseases can have several effects on disease development and progression. Here are some key effects:

Accelerated Cognitive Decline:

Elevated cortisol levels and chronic stress have been associated with accelerated cognitive decline in neurodegenerative diseases such as Alzheimer's disease. Prolonged exposure to high cortisol levels can contribute to the loss of synapses and the buildup of amyloid plaques and neurofibrillary tangles, hallmark features of Alzheimer's disease.

Aggravation of Motor Symptoms:

In neurodegenerative diseases involving movement disorders, such as Parkinson's disease and Huntington's disease, cortisol dysregulation can exacerbate motor symptoms. Elevated cortisol levels can worsen the severity of motor symptoms like tremors, rigidity, and bradykinesia, potentially impacting the quality of life for individuals with these conditions.

Neuroinflammation:

Cortisol dysregulation and chronic inflammation can contribute to neuroinflammation, a prominent feature in neurodegenerative diseases. Neuroinflammation involves the activation of immune cells in the brain, leading to the release of pro-inflammatory molecules. This sustained inflammatory response can exacerbate neuronal damage and accelerate disease progression.

Impact on Neuroprotective Mechanisms:

Cortisol dysregulation can interfere with the brain's natural neuroprotective mechanisms. For example, elevated cortisol levels can impair the clearance of toxic proteins, such as beta-amyloid in Alzheimer's disease, leading to their accumulation and subsequent neurodegeneration.

Managing Cortisol and Supporting Neurodegenerative Disease Management:

While the influence of cortisol on neurodegenerative diseases is complex, there are strategies that can be employed to manage cortisol levels and support disease management. Here are some recommendations:

Stress Reduction:

Engage in stress reduction techniques such as meditation, deep breathing exercises, yoga, or mindfulness practices. Chronic stress can contribute to cortisol dysregulation, exacerbating the progression of neurodegenerative diseases. By managing stress, cortisol levels can be regulated, potentially slowing disease progression, and enhancing overall well-being.

Cognitive Stimulation:

Engage in activities that stimulate the brain and promote cognitive function. Regular mental exercises, such as puzzles, reading, learning new skills, or participating in social activities, can help maintain cognitive abilities and potentially slow down cognitive decline in neurodegenerative diseases.

Healthy Lifestyle:

Adopt a healthy lifestyle that supports overall well-being. This includes eating a balanced diet rich in fruits, vegetables, whole grains, lean proteins, and healthy fats. Regular physical activity, adequate sleep, and maintaining social connections are also crucial. These lifestyle factors can contribute to overall health, support cortisol regulation, and potentially slow disease progression in neurodegenerative diseases.

Medication Management:

Work closely with healthcare professionals specializing in neurodegenerative diseases to develop an individualized medication plan. Medications may be prescribed to manage symptoms, slow disease progression, or target specific mechanisms involved in the disease process. Adhering to the prescribed medication regimen can help mitigate the impact of cortisol dysregulation on neurodegenerative diseases.

Supportive Care:

Incorporate supportive care interventions into the disease management plan. This may involve physical therapy, occupational therapy, speech therapy, or counseling services tailored to the specific needs of individuals with neurodegenerative diseases. Supportive care can enhance quality of life, improve functional abilities, and provide emotional support for individuals and their caregivers.

Ongoing Communication with Healthcare Professionals:

Maintain regular communication with healthcare professionals specializing in neurodegenerative diseases. They can provide guidance, monitor disease progression, adjust medications as needed, and offer support throughout the journey. Staying informed and actively involved in the management of the disease can make a significant difference in overall well-being.

So,

Cortisol, as a key player in the stress response, can influence the development and progression of neurodegenerative diseases. By understanding the complex relationship between cortisol and these diseases, individuals can make informed decisions about stress management, adopting a healthy lifestyle, engaging in cognitive stimulation, and seeking professional guidance when necessary.

While cortisol dysregulation can have a significant impact on neurodegenerative diseases, it's important to remember that the management of these conditions involves a multidimensional approach. By combining stress reduction techniques, a healthy lifestyle, medication management, supportive care, and ongoing communication with healthcare professionals, individuals can navigate the complexities of cortisol and neurodegenerative diseases while focusing on maintaining quality of life and well-being.

Chapter 38: The Impact of Chronic Noise and Loud Sounds on Cortisol Levels

We will explore the intriguing connection between cortisol levels and exposure to chronic noise or loud sounds. Cortisol, commonly known as the "stress hormone," plays a crucial role in our body's stress response and various physiological processes. Sound is an inherent part of our environment, but exposure to excessive or chronic noise can have profound effects on our well-being. In this chapter, we will delve into the details of how chronic noise and loud sounds can influence cortisol levels, shedding light on the mechanisms involved and offering insights into understanding and managing the impact of noise on our stress response.

Understanding Cortisol and the Stress Response:

Before we delve into the specifics of cortisol and noise exposure, let's establish a foundational understanding of these terms. Cortisol is a hormone produced by the adrenal glands in response to stress. It helps regulate various physiological processes, including metabolism, immune function, blood pressure, and inflammation. The stress response is the body's innate reaction to perceived threats or challenges, activating various physiological systems to prepare for action.

Cortisol's Influence on Noise Exposure:

Exposure to chronic noise or loud sounds can impact cortisol levels through several mechanisms. Here's a closer look at how noise influences the stress response and cortisol regulation:

Activation of the Sympathetic Nervous System:

When we encounter loud or persistent noise, it can trigger the activation of the sympathetic nervous system, which is responsible for the body's "fight-or-flight" response. This response involves the release of stress hormones, including cortisol, to prepare the body for immediate action. In this context, noise acts as a stressor that can elevate cortisol levels.

Sleep Disruption:

Chronic noise exposure, particularly during nighttime hours, can disrupt sleep patterns. Poor-quality sleep or sleep deprivation can lead to cortisol dysregulation, resulting in elevated cortisol levels. Sleep disturbance caused by noise can contribute to chronic stress and subsequent alterations in cortisol secretion.

Psychological and Perceived Stress:

Noise pollution can generate psychological stress and contribute to an overall sense of discomfort. Persistent exposure to loud sounds or chronic noise can evoke feelings of irritation, annoyance, and frustration, leading to increased perceived stress levels. Heightened psychological stress can trigger cortisol release, influencing cortisol levels.

Inflammatory Response:

Excessive or chronic noise exposure has been associated with increased inflammation in the body. Elevated cortisol levels, because of noise-induced stress, can modulate the immune system and potentially contribute to inflammation. Inflammatory processes may further impact cortisol regulation, creating a complex interplay between noise exposure, cortisol, and inflammation.

Effects of Noise Exposure on Cortisol Levels:

The impact of chronic noise or loud sounds on cortisol levels can have several effects on our well-being. Here are some key effects:

Increased Cortisol Levels:

Chronic exposure to noise or loud sounds can lead to elevated cortisol levels. Heightened cortisol levels are associated with various physiological changes in the body, such as increased blood pressure, altered metabolism, and impaired immune function. Prolonged elevation of cortisol can have detrimental effects on overall health if left unmanaged.

Stress-related Health Issues:

Prolonged elevation of cortisol due to chronic noise exposure can contribute to the development or exacerbation of stress-related health issues. These may include cardiovascular problems, digestive disorders, compromised immune function, sleep disturbances, and mental health conditions such as anxiety and depression. Cortisol dysregulation plays a significant role in the manifestation of these health issues.

Impact on Cognitive Function:

Elevated cortisol levels resulting from chronic noise exposure can affect cognitive function. Research suggests that chronic exposure to noise may impair attention, memory, learning, and problem-solving abilities. The disruptive effects of noise on cognitive function may be partially mediated by cortisol dysregulation.

Managing Noise Exposure and Cortisol Regulation:

To manage the impact of chronic noise or loud sounds on cortisol levels, it's important to consider strategies that minimize noise exposure and support a healthy stress response. Here are some recommendations:

Environmental Modifications:

Take steps to reduce noise levels in your environment. This may involve using soundproofing materials, installing double-glazed windows, or using white noise machines to mask background sounds. Creating a quiet and peaceful environment can help minimize chronic noise exposure and support cortisol regulation.

Time Spent in Quieter Settings:

Balance your time between noisy and quieter settings. Regularly seek out peaceful environments, such as nature reserves, parks, or quiet rooms, where you can escape the constant barrage of noise. Spending time in these serene spaces can help reduce stress levels and promote cortisol regulation.

Ear Protection:

When exposure to loud sounds is unavoidable, use ear protection measures such as earplugs or noise-canceling headphones. These devices can help reduce the intensity of sound and protect your ears from potential damage. By minimizing the impact of loud sounds on your auditory system, you can mitigate the stress response and potential cortisol dysregulation.

Stress Management Techniques:

Engage in stress reduction techniques to manage the impact of chronic noise exposure on cortisol levels. This may include practices such as meditation, deep breathing exercises, yoga, or engaging in hobbies and activities that promote relaxation. By managing stress levels, you can support cortisol regulation and promote overall well-being.

Sleep Hygiene:

Prioritize good sleep hygiene to counteract the effects of noise-induced sleep disruption. Create a sleep-friendly environment by using earplugs, white noise machines, or soothing sounds to mask disruptive noises. Establish consistent sleep routines, maintain a comfortable sleeping environment, and engage in relaxation techniques before bed to support restful sleep and cortisol regulation.

Healthy Lifestyle:

Adopt a healthy lifestyle that supports overall well-being and resilience to stress. This includes eating a balanced diet, engaging in regular physical activity, maintaining social connections, and practicing self-care. These lifestyle factors contribute to cortisol regulation and support the body's ability to cope with stress, including the stress induced by chronic noise exposure.

Mindfulness and Mental Wellness:

Incorporate mindfulness practices and prioritize mental wellness. Engaging in mindfulness-based stress reduction techniques, therapy, or counseling can help develop resilience to chronic noise exposure. By fostering mental well-being, you can enhance your ability to manage stress and maintain cortisol balance.

So,

Chronic noise exposure or exposure to loud sounds can have a significant impact on cortisol levels and overall well-being. By understanding the intricate relationship between noise and cortisol, individuals can take proactive steps to manage noise exposure, minimize its effects, and support cortisol regulation. Implementing environmental modifications, using ear protection, practicing stress management techniques, prioritizing sleep hygiene, adopting a healthy lifestyle, and cultivating mindfulness can all contribute to mitigating the impact of chronic noise exposure on cortisol levels.

Remember, the effects of noise on cortisol can vary among individuals, and it's important to find strategies that work best for you. By taking control of your environment, implementing stress reduction techniques, and prioritizing your well-being, you can navigate the challenges posed by chronic noise exposure while promoting a balanced stress response and cortisol regulation.

Chapter 39: Unraveling the Connection Between Cortisol and Appetite Regulation

We will explore the intriguing role of cortisol in regulating appetite and food cravings. Cortisol, commonly known as the "stress hormone," is a vital player in our body's stress response and various physiological processes. Appetite regulation, on the other hand, involves a complex interplay of hormones and signals that influence our desire for food and the sensation of hunger. In this chapter, we will delve into the details of how cortisol influences appetite and food cravings, shedding light on the mechanisms involved and offering insights into understanding and managing the effects of cortisol on our eating behaviors.

Understanding Cortisol and Appetite Regulation:

Before we delve into the specifics of cortisol and appetite, let's establish a foundational understanding of these terms. Cortisol is a hormone produced by the adrenal glands in response to stress. It helps regulate various physiological processes, including metabolism, immune function, blood pressure, and inflammation. Appetite regulation involves a network of hormones, neurotransmitters, and brain signals that control hunger, satiety, and food intake.

Cortisol's Influence on Appetite Regulation:

Cortisol can influence appetite regulation through various mechanisms. Here's a closer look at how cortisol interacts with our eating behaviors:

Stress-induced Changes in Appetite:

Cortisol levels rise in response to stress, and stress can have diverse effects on appetite. Some individuals experience a decrease in appetite during acute stress, while others may experience an increase in appetite, leading to stress eating. Cortisol, as a stress hormone, can impact the brain's reward and pleasure centers, influencing our desire for food and potentially leading to overeating or craving certain types of foods.

Regulation of Hunger and Satiety Hormones:

Cortisol interacts with other hormones involved in appetite regulation, including ghrelin and leptin. Ghrelin is often referred to as the "hunger hormone" because it stimulates appetite, while leptin is known as the "satiety hormone" as it signals fullness. Cortisol can modulate the production and sensitivity of these hormones, potentially influencing our feelings of hunger and satiety.

Impact on Food Preferences:

Cortisol can also influence our food preferences, especially during times of stress. Stress-induced cortisol release has been associated with a preference for energy-dense, highly palatable foods that are typically high in fat, sugar, or salt. These comfort foods can provide a temporary sense of relief or pleasure, leading to emotional eating and potential weight gain.

Emotional Eating:

Cortisol, in combination with other stress-related factors, can contribute to emotional eating. During times of stress, cortisol activates brain regions involved in emotional processing, such as the amygdala. This can lead to increased cravings for certain foods, particularly those that are associated with emotional comfort or reward.

Effects of Cortisol on Appetite Regulation:

The impact of cortisol on appetite regulation can have several effects on our eating behaviors and overall well-being. Here are some key effects:

Increased Food Intake:

Elevated cortisol levels, particularly in response to chronic stress, can contribute to an increase in food intake. This can lead to overeating or a preference for calorie-dense foods, potentially resulting in weight gain or difficulties in weight management.

Cravings for Unhealthy Foods:

Cortisol, when combined with emotional or psychological factors, can lead to cravings for unhealthy, comfort foods. These foods are often high in sugar, fat, or salt, providing a temporary sense of pleasure or relief. Frequent indulgence in such foods can have long-term implications for overall health and weight management.

Disrupted Eating Patterns:

Cortisol dysregulation can disrupt normal eating patterns. Some individuals may experience decreased appetite during times of stress, leading to inadequate food intake. Others may engage in emotional eating, using food as a coping mechanism to manage stress or emotional distress. Both scenarios can impact nutritional balance and overall well-being.

Managing Cortisol and Supporting Healthy Eating Habits:

To manage the impact of cortisol on appetite regulation and promote healthy eating habits, it's important to consider strategies that support cortisol regulation and mindful eating. Here are some recommendations:

Stress Management:

Engage in stress reduction techniques to manage cortisol levels and reduce stress-related eating behaviors. This may include activities such as meditation, deep breathing exercises, yoga, or engaging in hobbies that promote relaxation. By managing stress effectively, you can mitigate the impact of cortisol on appetite regulation.

Mindful Eating:

Practice mindful eating to develop a greater awareness of hunger and fullness cues, as well as the emotional factors influencing your eating behaviors. Mindful eating involves paying attention to the sensory aspects of food, eating slowly, and listening to your body's signals of hunger and satiety. By tuning into your body's needs, you can make conscious choices about when, what, and how much to eat.

Balanced Nutrition:

Focus on consuming a balanced diet that includes a variety of nutrient-rich foods. A well-rounded diet can help support overall health and minimize cravings for unhealthy foods. Include plenty of fruits, vegetables, whole grains, lean proteins, and healthy fats in your meals. These nutrient-dense foods provide essential vitamins, minerals, and antioxidants, promoting overall well-being.

Regular Meal Patterns:

Establish regular meal patterns and avoid skipping meals. Skipping meals can disrupt appetite regulation and lead to overeating or unhealthy food choices later in the day. Aim for balanced meals and snacks at regular intervals to maintain stable blood sugar levels and support consistent energy levels throughout the day.

Emotional Awareness:

Develop emotional awareness and alternative coping strategies for managing stress and emotions. Find healthy outlets for stress such as exercise, engaging in creative activities, spending time with loved ones, or seeking support from a therapist or counselor. By addressing emotional needs directly, you can reduce reliance on food as a means of emotional comfort.

Physical Activity:

Incorporate regular physical activity into your routine. Exercise has been shown to reduce cortisol levels, improve mood, and promote overall well-being. Engage in activities you enjoy, whether it's walking, dancing, swimming, or any form of exercise that brings you joy. Regular physical activity can help regulate cortisol levels and support healthy appetite regulation.

So,

Cortisol, as a key player in the stress response, can influence appetite regulation and food cravings. By understanding the complex relationship between cortisol and our eating behaviors, individuals can take proactive steps to manage cortisol levels, develop mindful eating habits, and promote overall well-being.

Implementing stress management techniques, practicing mindful eating, prioritizing balanced nutrition, establishing regular meal patterns, fostering emotional awareness, and engaging in regular physical activity can all contribute to mitigating the impact of cortisol on appetite regulation. Remember, healthy eating is a holistic endeavor that involves physical, emotional, and psychological factors. By nurturing a balanced approach to food and addressing stress in healthy ways, you can navigate the influence of cortisol on appetite and cultivate a positive relationship with food and your well-being.

Chapter 40: Unveiling the Impact of Cortisol on Vaccinations and Immunizations

We will explore the fascinating connection between cortisol and the body's response to vaccinations and immunizations. Cortisol, often referred to as the "stress hormone," plays a crucial role in our body's stress response and various physiological processes. Vaccinations and immunizations are essential tools in safeguarding our health by preventing infectious diseases. In this chapter, we will delve into the details of how cortisol influences the body's response to vaccinations, shedding light on the mechanisms involved and offering insights into understanding and optimizing the effectiveness of immunization strategies.

Understanding Cortisol and the Immune System:

Before we delve into the specifics of cortisol and vaccinations, let's establish a foundational understanding of these terms. Cortisol is a hormone produced by the adrenal glands in response to stress. It helps regulate various physiological processes, including metabolism, immune function, blood pressure, and inflammation. The immune system is a complex network of cells, tissues, and organs that work together to defend the body against harmful pathogens.

Cortisol's Influence on the Immune Response to Vaccinations:

Cortisol can influence the body's response to vaccinations through various mechanisms. Here's a closer look at how cortisol interacts with the immune system:

Immunomodulatory Effects:

Cortisol has immunomodulatory properties, meaning it can regulate immune responses. During times of stress, cortisol levels rise, and this elevation can impact the immune system. Elevated cortisol levels can suppress certain aspects of immune function, including the production of pro-inflammatory cytokines and the activity of immune cells such as lymphocytes. This immunosuppressive effect can potentially affect the body's response to vaccinations.

Impact on Vaccine-Induced Antibody Production:

Vaccinations stimulate the production of specific antibodies that provide protection against targeted pathogens. Cortisol can influence the production of these antibodies by affecting the activity of B cells, which are responsible for antibody production. Elevated cortisol levels have been associated with reduced antibody production in response to vaccines, potentially impacting their effectiveness.

Timing of Vaccinations:

Cortisol levels fluctuate throughout the day, with a natural peak in the morning and a gradual decline towards the evening. The timing of vaccinations in relation to cortisol rhythms may influence the immune response. Research suggests that vaccinations administered during periods of lower cortisol levels, such as in the morning, may result in a more robust immune response compared to vaccinations given during periods of higher cortisol levels.

Psychological Factors:

Stress and psychological factors can influence cortisol levels and, subsequently, the immune response to vaccinations. High levels of perceived stress, anxiety, or negative emotions can impact cortisol secretion, potentially affecting the immune system's ability to mount an optimal response to vaccines. Positive psychological states, on the other hand, may promote a more favorable immune response.

Effects of Cortisol on Vaccination Outcomes:

The impact of cortisol on the body's response to vaccinations can have several effects on immunization outcomes. Here are some key effects:

Vaccine Efficacy:

Elevated cortisol levels, particularly during periods of chronic stress, have been associated with decreased vaccine efficacy. The immunosuppressive effects of cortisol can impair the immune system's ability to generate a robust response to vaccines, potentially reducing the protective effect conferred by immunization.

Duration of Immunity:

Cortisol levels may also influence the duration of immunity provided by vaccinations. Lower cortisol levels, as observed during periods of lower stress or in the morning, have been associated with a longer duration of vaccine-induced immunity. Conversely, higher cortisol levels may contribute to a more rapid decline in vaccine-elicited protection.

Variability in Individual Responses:

Individual responses to vaccinations can vary due to multiple factors, including genetic variations, overall health, and stress levels. Cortisol levels, influenced by stress and other factors, may contribute to this variability in immune responses. Some individuals may experience a diminished response to vaccinations due to higher cortisol levels, while others may have a more robust response.

Potential Strategies for Optimization:

Understanding the influence of cortisol on vaccination outcomes can inform strategies for optimizing immunization effectiveness. Timing vaccinations during periods of lower cortisol levels, such as in the morning, may enhance the immune response. Additionally, managing stress and promoting psychological well-being through stress reduction techniques, mindfulness practices, and positive emotions may help modulate cortisol levels and support a more favorable immune response to vaccinations.

Managing Cortisol and Supporting Vaccine Responses:

While cortisol's influence on vaccination outcomes is a complex topic, there are strategies that can be employed to support optimal immune responses. Here are some recommendations:

Stress Reduction:

Engage in stress reduction techniques to manage cortisol levels and support a more favorable immune response to vaccinations. This may include practices such as meditation, deep breathing exercises, yoga, or engaging in activities that promote relaxation. By managing stress effectively, you can help mitigate the impact of cortisol on the immune system.

Optimal Timing of Vaccinations:

Consider the timing of vaccinations in relation to cortisol rhythms. Vaccinations administered during periods of lower cortisol levels, such as in the morning, may enhance the immune response. Discuss with healthcare professionals the possibility of scheduling vaccinations during these times when feasible.

Psychological Well-being:

Promote psychological well-being and positive emotions to support optimal immune responses. Engage in activities that promote positive mental states, such as practicing gratitude, engaging in hobbies, connecting with loved ones, and seeking emotional support when needed. These factors can help modulate cortisol levels and support a more favorable immune response to vaccines.

Adherence to Vaccination Schedules:

Ensure adherence to recommended vaccination schedules. Following the recommended immunization timelines is essential for establishing optimal protection against infectious diseases. Consult healthcare professionals for guidance on the appropriate vaccination schedule for you and your loved ones.

Healthy Lifestyle:

Adopt a healthy lifestyle that supports overall immune function. This includes eating a balanced diet rich in fruits, vegetables, whole grains, lean proteins, and healthy fats. Engage in regular physical activity, get adequate sleep, and practice good hygiene to support overall health and immune system function.

Open Communication with Healthcare Professionals:

Maintain open communication with healthcare professionals regarding any concerns or questions about vaccinations. They can provide guidance, address any specific considerations related to cortisol and vaccination responses, and offer personalized recommendations based on individual circumstances.

So,

Cortisol, as a key player in the stress response, can influence the body's response to vaccinations. By understanding the complex relationship between cortisol and immunization outcomes, individuals can take proactive steps to manage stress, optimize timing, and support the immune response to vaccines.

Implementing stress reduction techniques, considering optimal timing for vaccinations, fostering psychological well-being, adhering to vaccination schedules, maintaining a healthy lifestyle, and engaging in open communication with healthcare professionals can all contribute to mitigating the impact of cortisol on vaccine responses.

Remember, vaccinations are vital for protecting our health and preventing the spread of infectious diseases. By optimizing our immune responses to vaccines and managing cortisol levels, we can play an active role in safeguarding our well-being and the health of our communities.

Chapter 41: The Intricate Connection Between Cortisol and Metabolic Syndrome

We will explore the fascinating link between cortisol and the development and progression of metabolic syndrome. Cortisol, commonly known as the "stress hormone," plays a vital role in our body's stress response and various physiological processes. Metabolic syndrome is a cluster of interconnected conditions that increase the risk of developing cardiovascular disease, type 2 diabetes, and other health complications. In this chapter, we will delve into the details of how cortisol influences metabolic syndrome, shedding light on the mechanisms involved and offering insights into understanding and managing its impact on our metabolic health.

Understanding Cortisol and Metabolic Syndrome:

Before we delve into the specifics of cortisol and metabolic syndrome, let's establish a foundational understanding of these terms. Cortisol is a hormone produced by the adrenal glands in response to stress. It helps regulate various physiological processes, including metabolism, immune function, blood pressure, and inflammation. Metabolic syndrome is a term used to describe a cluster of conditions, including abdominal obesity, high blood pressure, high blood sugar levels, abnormal lipid levels, and insulin resistance, that collectively increase the risk of developing chronic diseases.

Cortisol's Influence on Metabolic Syndrome:

Cortisol can influence the development and progression of metabolic syndrome through various mechanisms. Here's a closer look at how cortisol interacts with metabolic health:

Abdominal Fat Accumulation:

Cortisol has been implicated in the accumulation of abdominal fat, which is a key characteristic of metabolic syndrome. Elevated cortisol levels, particularly because of chronic stress, can lead to an increase in visceral adipose tissue (fat around the abdominal organs). This type of fat is metabolically active and associated with insulin resistance, inflammation, and other factors contributing to metabolic syndrome.

Insulin Resistance:

Insulin resistance is a hallmark of metabolic syndrome, characterized by decreased responsiveness of cells to the hormone insulin. Cortisol can impair insulin sensitivity, making it more difficult for cells to take up glucose from the bloodstream. This can lead to elevated blood sugar levels and an increased risk of developing type 2 diabetes.

Dysregulation of Glucose Metabolism:

Cortisol plays a role in regulating glucose metabolism. It promotes the breakdown of glycogen (stored glucose) in the liver and stimulates glucose production through a process called gluconeogenesis. Chronically elevated cortisol levels can disrupt the delicate balance of glucose regulation, potentially contributing to metabolic dysfunction.

Disruption of Lipid Metabolism:

Cortisol can also influence lipid metabolism, including the production and breakdown of fats. Elevated cortisol levels have been associated with increased levels of triglycerides (a type of fat) and decreased levels of high-density lipoprotein (HDL) cholesterol, commonly known as "good" cholesterol. These lipid abnormalities contribute to the lipid profile seen in metabolic syndrome.

Blood Pressure Regulation:

Chronic stress and elevated cortisol levels can impact blood pressure regulation. Cortisol can increase blood pressure by promoting vasoconstriction (narrowing of blood vessels) and enhancing the effects of other blood pressure-regulating hormones, such as angiotensin II. Elevated blood pressure is a key component of metabolic syndrome and contributes to cardiovascular risk.

Effects of Cortisol on Metabolic Syndrome:

The impact of cortisol on metabolic syndrome can have several effects on overall metabolic health. Here are some key effects:

Increased Risk of Developing Metabolic Syndrome:

Chronic elevation of cortisol levels, particularly because of chronic stress, is associated with an increased risk of developing metabolic syndrome. The interplay between cortisol and metabolic processes, including abdominal fat accumulation, insulin resistance, dysregulated glucose and lipid metabolism, and elevated blood pressure, can contribute to the development and progression of metabolic syndrome.

Aggravation of Existing Metabolic Syndrome:

Elevated cortisol levels can exacerbate the metabolic dysfunction seen in individuals already diagnosed with metabolic syndrome. Cortisol's influence on insulin sensitivity, lipid metabolism, and blood pressure regulation can further contribute to the progression of metabolic abnormalities and increase the risk of complications such as cardiovascular disease and type 2 diabetes.

Impact on Weight Management:

Cortisol dysregulation can impact weight management efforts. Elevated cortisol levels, particularly in response to chronic stress, have been associated with increased appetite, cravings for high-calorie foods, and the redistribution of fat to the abdominal region. These factors can make it more challenging to achieve and maintain a healthy weight, further contributing to metabolic syndrome.

Managing Cortisol and Promoting Metabolic Health:

While cortisol's influence on metabolic syndrome is complex, there are strategies that can be employed to manage cortisol levels and promote metabolic health. Here are some recommendations:

Stress Management:

Engage in stress reduction techniques to manage cortisol levels and promote metabolic health. This may include practices such as meditation, deep breathing exercises, yoga, regular physical activity, and engaging in hobbies or activities that promote relaxation. By managing stress effectively, you can help mitigate the impact of cortisol on metabolic processes.

Healthy Lifestyle:

Adopt a healthy lifestyle that supports overall metabolic health. This includes following a balanced diet rich in whole foods, such as fruits, vegetables, whole grains, lean proteins, and healthy fats. Regular physical activity, adequate sleep, and maintaining a healthy weight are also key components of a metabolic-healthy lifestyle.

Regular Exercise:

Incorporate regular exercise into your routine. Physical activity can help regulate cortisol levels, improve insulin sensitivity, promote weight management, and enhance overall metabolic health. Aim for a combination of aerobic exercises, strength training, and flexibility exercises to achieve comprehensive benefits.

Balanced Nutrition:

Focus on balanced nutrition to support metabolic health. Avoid excessive consumption of processed foods, sugary beverages, and high-fat foods. Instead, emphasize nutrient-dense, whole foods that provide essential vitamins, minerals, fiber, and antioxidants. Consult with healthcare professionals or registered dietitians for personalized guidance on optimizing your nutritional intake.

Sleep Hygiene:

Prioritize good sleep hygiene to support cortisol regulation and metabolic health. Aim for adequate and restful sleep by establishing a consistent sleep schedule, creating a relaxing bedtime routine, optimizing your sleep environment, and avoiding stimulants like caffeine close to bedtime. Quality sleep promotes hormonal balance and supports metabolic processes.

Regular Health Check-ups:

Schedule regular check-ups with healthcare professionals to monitor your metabolic health. Regular monitoring of blood pressure, blood sugar levels, lipid profiles, and other relevant markers can help identify any early signs of metabolic dysfunction. Collaborate with healthcare professionals to develop personalized strategies for managing and improving metabolic health.

So,

Cortisol, as a key player in the stress response, can influence the development and progression of metabolic syndrome. By understanding the complex relationship between cortisol and metabolic health, individuals can take proactive steps to manage stress, optimize lifestyle choices, and promote metabolic well-being.

Implementing stress reduction techniques, adopting a healthy lifestyle, engaging in regular exercise, focusing on balanced nutrition, prioritizing quality sleep, and maintaining regular health check-ups are all integral components of managing cortisol levels and supporting metabolic health.

Remember, metabolic syndrome is a multifaceted condition influenced by various factors. By making positive changes and seeking appropriate guidance, you can take control of your metabolic health and reduce the risk of complications associated with metabolic syndrome.

Chapter 42: Unraveling the Relationship Between Cortisol and Hormonal Contraceptives

We will explore the intriguing connection between cortisol levels and hormonal contraceptives. Cortisol, commonly known as the "stress hormone," is a key player in our body's stress response and various physiological processes. Hormonal contraceptives, on the other hand, are widely used methods of birth control that contain synthetic hormones. In this chapter, we will delve into the details of how hormonal contraceptives can influence cortisol levels, shedding light on the mechanisms involved and offering insights into understanding the interplay between these two factors.

Understanding Cortisol and Hormonal Contraceptives:

Before we delve into the specifics of cortisol and hormonal contraceptives, let's establish a foundational understanding of these terms. Cortisol is a hormone produced by the adrenal glands in response to stress. It plays a crucial role in various physiological processes, including metabolism, immune function, blood pressure regulation, and inflammation. Hormonal contraceptives, such as birth control pills, patches, injections, and hormonal intrauterine devices (IUDs), contain synthetic hormones that prevent pregnancy by inhibiting ovulation or altering the uterine lining.

Cortisol's Interaction with Hormonal Contraceptives:

Hormonal contraceptives can influence cortisol levels through various mechanisms. Here's a closer look at how cortisol and hormonal contraceptives interact:

Estrogen and Progestin Effects:

Hormonal contraceptives, particularly combined hormonal contraceptives that contain both estrogen and progestin, can impact cortisol levels. Estrogen has been found to increase cortisol-binding globulin (CBG), a protein that binds to cortisol in the bloodstream. This can lead to higher levels of CBG-bound cortisol, potentially influencing the availability and activity of free cortisol.

Progestin Influence:

Progestin, a synthetic form of the hormone progesterone, is a key component of hormonal contraceptives. Different progestin types can have varying effects on cortisol levels. Some progestins have been found to increase cortisol levels, while others have shown no significant impact. The specific progestin used in a particular hormonal contraceptive can influence its effect on cortisol.

Stress and Cortisol Response:

Stress can influence cortisol levels, and hormonal contraceptives may modulate the body's response to stress. Some studies suggest that women using hormonal contraceptives may have blunted cortisol responses to stress compared to non-users. This blunted response may be attributed to the hormonal effects of contraceptives, but further research is needed to fully understand the mechanisms involved.

Effects of Hormonal Contraceptives on Cortisol Levels:

The impact of hormonal contraceptives on cortisol levels can have several effects. Here are some key considerations:

Cortisol Binding:

Hormonal contraceptives, particularly those containing estrogen, can increase the levels of CBG-bound cortisol. This can potentially affect the availability and activity of free cortisol, which is the biologically active form. The overall impact on cortisol function and stress response requires further investigation.

Cortisol Metabolism:

Hormonal contraceptives may also influence cortisol metabolism. Some studies suggest that progestins used in hormonal contraceptives can alter the enzymes involved in cortisol metabolism, potentially affecting cortisol clearance rates. This, in turn, can influence cortisol levels and dynamics in the body.

Emotional Well-being:

Cortisol is intricately linked to emotional well-being, and hormonal contraceptives can influence mood and emotions. Some individuals may experience changes in mood, including symptoms of anxiety or depression, while using hormonal contraceptives. The specific impact on cortisol levels and its contribution to emotional well-being requires further research.

Individual Variability:

It's important to note that individual responses to hormonal contraceptives can vary. While some individuals may experience changes in cortisol levels or stress response while using hormonal contraceptives, others may not observe significant differences. Factors such as overall health, genetics, lifestyle, and stress levels can contribute to individual variability in cortisol responses.

Considerations for Hormonal Contraceptive Users:

If you are using or considering using hormonal contraceptives, here are some important considerations:

Consult with Healthcare Professionals:

Discuss any concerns or questions about hormonal contraceptives with healthcare professionals. They can provide personalized guidance based on your specific health profile and help you make informed decisions regarding contraception.

Monitoring Cortisol Levels:

If you have specific concerns about cortisol levels or stress response while using hormonal contraceptives, consider discussing the option of cortisol testing with healthcare professionals. This can provide insights into your individual cortisol dynamics and guide any necessary adjustments or interventions.

Awareness of Emotional Well-being:

Be mindful of your emotional well-being while using hormonal contraceptives. If you notice significant changes in mood or emotions, discuss these changes with healthcare professionals. They can help determine if these changes are related to hormonal contraceptives or if there may be other factors contributing to your emotional well-being.

Managing Stress:

Stress management is important for overall well-being, regardless of contraceptive use. Engage in stress reduction techniques, such as mindfulness practices, exercise, and seeking social support. These strategies can help mitigate the impact of stress on cortisol levels and promote overall health.

So,

Hormonal contraceptives can potentially influence cortisol levels, although the exact mechanisms and implications require further research. Estrogen and progestin components of hormonal contraceptives may affect cortisol binding, metabolism, and stress response. Individual responses to hormonal contraceptives can vary, and monitoring emotional well-being and stress levels is important.

If you have specific concerns about cortisol levels or stress response while using hormonal contraceptives, consult with healthcare professionals for personalized guidance. Remember that hormonal contraceptives provide effective contraception and play a crucial role in family planning. By staying informed and working closely with healthcare professionals, you can make informed decisions and optimize your reproductive health.

Chapter 43: Cortisol's Influence on Liver Function and Detoxification Processes

We will explore the intriguing impact of cortisol on liver function and detoxification processes. Cortisol, commonly known as the "stress hormone," plays a crucial role in our body's stress response and various physiological processes. The liver, on the other hand, is a remarkable organ responsible for numerous vital functions, including metabolism, detoxification, and the production of essential substances. In this chapter, we will delve into the details of how cortisol influences liver function and the intricate processes of detoxification, shedding light on their interplay and offering insights into understanding and supporting liver health.

Understanding Cortisol and the Liver:

Before we delve into the specifics of cortisol and its impact on the liver, let's establish a foundational understanding of these terms. Cortisol is a hormone produced by the adrenal glands in response to stress. It helps regulate various physiological processes, including metabolism, immune function, blood pressure regulation, and inflammation. The liver, one of the largest organs in the body, performs a wide range of critical functions, such as metabolizing nutrients, synthesizing proteins, storing vitamins and minerals, and detoxifying harmful substances.

Cortisol's Influence on Liver Function:

Cortisol can impact liver function through various mechanisms. Here's a closer look at how cortisol and the liver interact:

Gluconeogenesis and Glycogen Metabolism:

Cortisol stimulates the process of gluconeogenesis, which is the production of glucose from non-carbohydrate sources, primarily amino acids. The liver plays a significant role in this process, and cortisol's influence can increase glucose production and release into the bloodstream. Additionally, cortisol promotes the breakdown of glycogen, the stored form of glucose, in the liver. These actions help maintain adequate blood glucose levels during times of stress.

Lipid Metabolism:

Cortisol can affect lipid metabolism in the liver. It promotes the breakdown of fats through lipolysis, leading to increased fatty acid release into the bloodstream. These fatty acids can be utilized for energy production or stored as body fat. Cortisol can also influence the synthesis and breakdown of cholesterol in the liver, which plays a vital role in various physiological processes.

Protein Metabolism:

Cortisol affects protein metabolism in the liver by promoting protein breakdown, or proteolysis. This process provides amino acids that can be used for gluconeogenesis or other metabolic processes. Cortisol's influence on protein metabolism helps provide necessary building blocks for energy production during stressful periods.

Inflammation and Immune Response:

The liver is an essential component of the immune system, playing a role in the detection and clearance of pathogens and toxins. Cortisol has anti-inflammatory properties and can suppress immune responses. While this modulation of inflammation can be beneficial in some situations, chronic elevation of cortisol levels may lead to impaired immune function and liver health.

Effects of Cortisol on Detoxification Processes:

The liver is responsible for detoxifying harmful substances that enter our bodies. Cortisol can influence these detoxification processes. Here are some key considerations:

Phase I Detoxification:

Phase I detoxification is the first step in the liver's detoxification process. It involves enzymes called cytochrome P450 (CYP) enzymes, which help convert toxins into intermediate forms for further processing. Cortisol can influence the activity of these enzymes, potentially impacting the speed and efficiency of phase I detoxification.

Phase II Detoxification:

Phase II detoxification involves the conjugation of toxins with molecules such as glutathione, sulfate, or glucuronic acid, making them more water-soluble and easier to eliminate from the body. Cortisol can modulate the activity of enzymes involved in phase II detoxification processes. Imbalances in cortisol levels may affect the liver's ability to efficiently process and eliminate toxins.

Bile Production:

Bile, produced by the liver, plays a vital role in the digestion and elimination of dietary fats and the excretion of waste products. Cortisol can influence bile production and the flow of bile from the liver into the gallbladder and intestines. This, in turn, can affect the absorption and elimination of toxins and waste products from the body.

Oxidative Stress:

Chronic elevation of cortisol levels, particularly as a result of chronic stress, can contribute to oxidative stress in the liver. Oxidative stress occurs when there is an imbalance between the production of reactive oxygen species (ROS) and the body's antioxidant defenses. Prolonged oxidative stress can damage liver cells and impair their detoxification capacity.

Supporting Liver Health and Detoxification:

Maintaining optimal liver health and supporting detoxification processes is crucial for overall well-being. Here are some recommendations:

Balanced Nutrition:

Follow a balanced diet that supports liver health. Include a variety of fruits, vegetables, whole grains, lean proteins, and healthy fats in your diet. Limit the consumption of processed foods, ..., and substances that can burden the liver, such as excessive sugar, unhealthy fats, and artificial additives.

Hydration:

Stay adequately hydrated to support liver function and detoxification processes. Water helps transport toxins and waste products out of the body. Aim to drink sufficient water throughout the day and limit the consumption of sugary beverages and excessive caffeine, which can place additional stress on the liver.

Limit ... Consumption:

Excessive ... consumption can have detrimental effects on the liver. Limit ... intake or avoid it altogether to support liver health and minimize the risk of liver damage.

Manage Stress:

Chronic stress can impact cortisol levels and liver health. Engage in stress reduction techniques, such as mindfulness practices, exercise, and seeking social support. By managing stress effectively, you can help mitigate the impact of cortisol on liver function and support overall liver health.

Regular Exercise:

Engage in regular physical activity to support liver health and overall well-being. Exercise promotes blood circulation, which helps deliver oxygen and nutrients to the liver. It also supports healthy metabolism and weight management, reducing the burden on the liver.

Minimize Toxin Exposure:

Limit exposure to environmental toxins whenever possible. This includes reducing exposure to pollutants, chemicals, and other harmful substances that can burden the liver. Consider using natural and eco-friendly products, optimizing indoor air quality, and adopting lifestyle choices that minimize exposure to toxins.

So,

Cortisol, as a key hormone in our stress response, can impact liver function and the intricate processes of detoxification. Understanding the interplay between cortisol and the liver provides insights into supporting liver health and optimizing detoxification processes.

By adopting a balanced nutrition plan, staying hydrated, limiting ... consumption, managing stress effectively, engaging in regular exercise, and minimizing toxin exposure, you can support liver health and facilitate efficient detoxification. Remember, the liver is a remarkable organ with incredible regenerative abilities. By taking proactive steps to support its health, you contribute to your overall well-being and vitality.

Chapter 44: The Intricate Dance Between Cortisol and Fasting/Calorie Restriction

We will dive into the fascinating relationship between cortisol and the body's response to fasting and calorie restriction. Cortisol, commonly known as the "stress hormone," plays a vital role in our body's stress response and various physiological processes. Fasting and calorie restriction, on the other hand, are dietary practices that involve periods of reduced or no food intake. In this chapter, we will explore how cortisol influences the body's response to fasting and calorie restriction, shedding light on the mechanisms involved and offering insights into understanding and optimizing these practices for health and well-being.

Understanding Cortisol and Fasting/Calorie Restriction:

Before we delve into the specifics of cortisol and its impact on fasting and calorie restriction, let's establish a foundational understanding of these terms. Cortisol is a hormone produced by the adrenal glands in response to stress. It helps regulate various physiological processes, including metabolism, immune function, blood pressure regulation, and inflammation. Fasting involves voluntarily abstaining from food for a specified period, while calorie restriction refers to reducing caloric intake below normal levels for weight management or health purposes.

Cortisol's Influence on the Body's Response to Fasting and Calorie Restriction:

Cortisol can influence the body's response to fasting and calorie restriction through various mechanisms. Here's a closer look at how cortisol and these dietary practices interact:

Glucose Regulation:

Cortisol plays a crucial role in maintaining glucose levels during fasting and calorie restriction. When the body is deprived of food, cortisol helps mobilize glucose from glycogen stores in the liver (glycogenolysis) and promotes the production of glucose from non-carbohydrate sources (gluconeogenesis). These processes ensure a steady supply of glucose to meet the body's energy needs.

Energy Conservation:

During fasting or calorie restriction, cortisol helps the body conserve energy by promoting the breakdown of stored fats (lipolysis) and sparing glucose for vital functions, such as brain activity and red blood cell production. This metabolic shift allows the body to utilize fatty acids as an alternative fuel source, helping to preserve glucose for essential processes.

Muscle Protein Breakdown:

In prolonged fasting or severe calorie restriction, cortisol can contribute to muscle protein breakdown (proteolysis) to provide amino acids for gluconeogenesis. This breakdown helps supply the body with glucose when glycogen stores are depleted. However, this effect can be minimized by maintaining adequate protein intake during fasting or calorie restriction.

Metabolic Adaptation:

Cortisol is involved in the body's metabolic adaptation to fasting and calorie restriction. When caloric intake is reduced, cortisol levels tend to increase to help regulate metabolism and conserve energy. This adaptation involves a decrease in resting metabolic rate, which helps the body adjust to the reduced caloric intake and promote energy conservation.

Stress Response:

Fasting and calorie restriction can be perceived as stressors by the body, leading to an increase in cortisol production. This stress response can influence various physiological processes, including immune function, inflammation, and the release of other hormones involved in the stress response. However, the degree of cortisol increases during fasting, or calorie restriction may vary depending on individual factors, such as overall health, stress levels, and duration of fasting or calorie restriction.

Effects of Cortisol on Fasting and Calorie Restriction:

Understanding the effects of cortisol on fasting and calorie restriction can provide insights into optimizing these practices for health and well-being. Here are some key considerations:

Glucose Availability:

Cortisol helps maintain glucose availability during fasting and calorie restriction. However, prolonged elevation of cortisol levels, particularly as a result of chronic stress, can contribute to insulin resistance and impaired glucose metabolism. Therefore, it is essential to strike a balance between cortisol-mediated glucose regulation and long-term metabolic health.

Muscle Preservation:

While cortisol can contribute to muscle protein breakdown during fasting or calorie restriction, adequate protein intake and resistance exercise can help mitigate muscle loss. Including high-quality protein sources in meals and engaging in strength training exercises can support muscle preservation and overall body composition during periods of reduced caloric intake.

Individual Variability:

Individual responses to fasting and calorie restriction, including cortisol levels and metabolic adaptations, can vary. Factors such as overall health, genetics, stress levels, and duration of fasting or calorie restriction can influence these responses. It is crucial to listen to your body, monitor your well-being, and consult with healthcare professionals or registered dietitians for personalized guidance.

Stress Management:

As fasting and calorie restriction can induce physiological and psychological stress, managing stress effectively is important. Engaging in stress reduction techniques, such as mindfulness practices, relaxation exercises, and adequate sleep, can help mitigate the impact of stress on cortisol levels and promote overall well-being during these dietary practices.

Balanced Nutrition:

When practicing fasting or calorie restriction, it's important to focus on nutrient-dense foods to support overall health. During eating windows or mealtimes, include a variety of fruits, vegetables, whole grains, lean proteins, and healthy fats to ensure adequate nutrient intake. This helps support the body's nutritional needs and optimize metabolic processes.

So,

Cortisol, as a key hormone involved in the stress response, can influence the body's response to fasting and calorie restriction. Understanding the interplay between cortisol and these dietary practices provides insights into optimizing their effects on health and well-being.

By maintaining a balanced approach to fasting or calorie restriction, including adequate protein intake, engaging in resistance exercise, managing stress effectively, and prioritizing nutrient-dense foods, you can support your body's response to these practices. Remember, individual responses may vary, and it's essential to listen to your body, monitor your well-being, and consult with healthcare professionals or registered dietitians for personalized guidance on incorporating fasting or calorie restriction into your lifestyle.

Chapter 45: Unveiling the Connection Between Cortisol and Gastrointestinal Disorders

We will explore the intriguing relationship between cortisol and gastrointestinal disorders. Cortisol, commonly known as the "stress hormone," plays a vital role in our body's stress response and various physiological processes. Gastrointestinal disorders encompass a wide range of conditions affecting the digestive system, including irritable bowel syndrome (IBS), inflammatory bowel disease (IBD), acid reflux, and others. In this chapter, we will delve into the details of how cortisol influences the development and progression of gastrointestinal disorders, shedding light on the mechanisms involved and offering insights into understanding and managing these conditions.

Understanding Cortisol and Gastrointestinal Disorders:

Before we dive into the specifics of cortisol and its impact on gastrointestinal disorders, let's establish a foundational understanding of these terms. Cortisol is a hormone produced by the adrenal glands in response to stress. It helps regulate various physiological processes, including metabolism, immune function, blood pressure regulation, and inflammation. Gastrointestinal disorders encompass a range of conditions affecting the digestive system, characterized by symptoms such as abdominal pain, diarrhea, constipation, bloating, and changes in bowel habits.

Cortisol's Influence on Gastrointestinal Disorders:

Cortisol can influence gastrointestinal disorders through various mechanisms. Here's a closer look at how cortisol and these conditions interact:

Stress and Gut-Brain Axis:

The gut-brain axis is a bidirectional communication network between the gastrointestinal system and the brain. Cortisol, as a key stress hormone, can impact this axis. Psychological and physical stressors can trigger cortisol release, which can affect the function and sensitivity of the gastrointestinal tract. Increased cortisol levels may contribute to gastrointestinal symptoms, including alterations in bowel movements, increased gut permeability, and heightened sensitivity to pain.

Immune System Modulation:

Cortisol has immunomodulatory effects that can influence the development and progression of gastrointestinal disorders. In conditions such as IBD, where the immune system plays a significant role, cortisol can dampen immune responses and reduce inflammation. However, chronic, or excessive cortisol levels can impair immune function and compromise the body's ability to manage inflammation, potentially exacerbating gastrointestinal symptoms.

Gut Motility and Sensitivity:

Cortisol can influence gut motility, or the movement of food through the digestive system. Stress-related cortisol release may contribute to changes in gut motility, leading to symptoms such as diarrhea or constipation. Additionally, cortisol can affect gut sensitivity, potentially amplifying pain signals and increasing the perception of discomfort or abdominal pain in individuals with gastrointestinal disorders.

Gut Microbiota:

The gut microbiota, a community of microorganisms in the digestive system, plays a crucial role in gastrointestinal health. Cortisol can influence the composition and diversity of the gut microbiota. Stress-induced cortisol release may alter the balance of beneficial and harmful bacteria, potentially impacting gut health and contributing to gastrointestinal symptoms.

Effects of Cortisol on Gastrointestinal Disorders:

Understanding the effects of cortisol on gastrointestinal disorders can provide insights into managing these conditions. Here are some key considerations:

Stress Management:

Given the influence of stress on cortisol release and gastrointestinal symptoms, stress management techniques are crucial in managing gastrointestinal disorders. Engaging in stress reduction practices such as mindfulness, relaxation exercises, regular physical activity, and seeking social support can help modulate cortisol levels and alleviate symptoms.

Dietary Modifications:

Diet plays a significant role in gastrointestinal health. While cortisol itself does not directly cause gastrointestinal disorders, stress-induced cortisol release may affect dietary choices and eating patterns, potentially aggravating symptoms. Adopting a well-balanced diet that includes fiber-rich foods, probiotics, and adequate hydration can support digestive health and minimize symptom flare-ups.

Sleep Quality:

Quality sleep is essential for overall well-being, including gastrointestinal health. Cortisol levels follow a diurnal pattern, with the highest levels in the morning and the lowest in the evening. Disruptions in the sleep-wake cycle and inadequate sleep can affect cortisol regulation and potentially impact gastrointestinal symptoms. Prioritizing good sleep hygiene practices can help maintain a healthy cortisol rhythm and support digestive health.

Mind-Body Techniques:

Mind-body techniques, such as meditation, deep breathing exercises, and yoga, can help reduce stress levels and promote relaxation. These practices have been shown to modulate cortisol levels and improve gastrointestinal symptoms in some individuals. Integrating mind-body techniques into daily routines may offer benefits in managing gastrointestinal disorders.

Medication and Therapy:

For individuals with more severe gastrointestinal disorders, healthcare professionals may recommend medications or therapy options to manage symptoms and improve overall well-being. These treatments are tailored to the specific condition and may include anti-inflammatory medications, antispasmodics, antidepressants, or therapies such as cognitive-behavioral therapy (CBT) to address stress and emotional factors.

So,

Cortisol, as a key hormone in our stress response, can influence the development and progression of gastrointestinal disorders. Understanding the interplay between cortisol and these conditions provides insights into managing symptoms and promoting gastrointestinal health.

By adopting stress management techniques, implementing dietary modifications, prioritizing quality sleep, incorporating mind-body practices, and working closely with healthcare professionals, individuals can develop personalized strategies to manage gastrointestinal disorders. Remember, each person's experience with gastrointestinal disorders is unique, and it is essential to seek professional guidance for an accurate diagnosis and tailored treatment plan. With proactive management and support, it is possible to alleviate symptoms and improve overall gastrointestinal health.

Chapter 46: Unraveling the Connection Between Cortisol and Infections

We will explore the intriguing relationship between cortisol and infections. Cortisol, commonly known as the "stress hormone," plays a crucial role in our body's stress response and various physiological processes. Infections, caused by pathogens such as bacteria, viruses, fungi, or parasites, can trigger immune responses to fight off invading microorganisms. In this chapter, we will delve into the details of how cortisol levels can be influenced by certain types of infections, shedding light on the mechanisms involved and offering insights into understanding the complex interplay between cortisol and the immune system during infection.

Understanding Cortisol and Infections:

Before we dive into the specifics of cortisol and its connection to infections, let's establish a foundational understanding of these terms. Cortisol is a hormone produced by the adrenal glands in response to stress. It helps regulate various physiological processes, including metabolism, immune function, blood pressure regulation, and inflammation. Infections occur when microorganisms invade the body, leading to immune responses aimed at neutralizing and eliminating the pathogens.

Cortisol's Influence on the Immune Response to Infections:

Cortisol can impact the immune response to infections through various mechanisms. Here's a closer look at how cortisol and infections interact:

Stress and Cortisol Release:

Infections can induce a stress response in the body, triggering the release of cortisol. This response is part of the body's defense mechanism to mobilize resources and support immune function during infection. Cortisol helps regulate inflammation, modulate immune cell activity, and maintain homeostasis.

Immune System Modulation:

Cortisol has immunomodulatory effects that can influence the immune response to infections. During infection, cortisol can suppress certain aspects of the immune system to prevent excessive inflammation and tissue damage. This regulatory role helps maintain a balanced immune response, allowing the body to effectively combat the infection while minimizing potential harm to the host.

Anti-inflammatory Effects:

Infections often lead to an inflammatory response as part of the immune system's defense mechanism. Cortisol has potent anti-inflammatory properties that can help control and resolve inflammation. By inhibiting the production of pro-inflammatory molecules, such as cytokines, cortisol plays a crucial role in dampening the immune response and preventing excessive inflammation.

Immune Cell Function:

Cortisol can influence the activity and function of immune cells involved in the immune response to infections. For instance, cortisol can reduce the activity of certain immune cells, such as T cells and natural killer (NK) cells, which are responsible for detecting and eliminating infected cells. This modulation helps prevent hyperactivation of the immune system and potential tissue damage.

Effects of Cortisol on Infection Outcome:

Understanding the effects of cortisol on infections can provide insights into the body's response and potential implications for infection outcome. Here are some key considerations:

Immunocompromised States:

Excessive or prolonged elevation of cortisol levels, such as in chronic stress or certain medical conditions, can lead to immunosuppression. This state can weaken the immune response to infections, making individuals more susceptible to microbial invasion and impairing the ability to effectively combat pathogens. It is important to manage stress levels and maintain a healthy cortisol balance to support immune function during infections.

Severity and Duration of Infection:

The interplay between cortisol and infections can influence the severity and duration of the infection. While cortisol's anti-inflammatory effects can help limit tissue damage and inflammation, excessive or prolonged cortisol release may hinder the immune system's ability to clear the infection efficiently. Striking a balance between cortisol modulation and an effective immune response is crucial for infection resolution.

Recovery and Healing:

Cortisol levels tend to normalize as the infection is resolved, allowing the immune system to return to its balanced state. However, in certain cases, prolonged elevation of cortisol levels or dysregulation of the stress response may delay healing and hinder recovery from infections. Supporting stress management and ensuring adequate rest, nutrition, and hydration can contribute to a healthy recovery process.

Individual Variability:

The interplay between cortisol and infections can vary among individuals. Factors such as overall health, genetic predispositions, previous exposure to similar pathogens, and lifestyle factors can influence the immune response and cortisol modulation during infections. It is important to remember that everyone's immune system and stress response are unique, and individual experiences with infections may differ.

So,

Cortisol, as a key hormone involved in the stress response, plays a complex role in the immune response to infections. Understanding the interplay between cortisol and infections provides insights into the body's defense mechanisms and potential implications for infection outcomes.

By managing stress levels, adopting healthy lifestyle practices, ensuring adequate rest and nutrition, and seeking appropriate medical care, individuals can support their immune system's response to infections. It is essential to prioritize overall well-being and consult with healthcare professionals for guidance on managing infections, especially in cases of chronic or severe infections. With a balanced approach, it is possible to optimize the body's immune response and support a healthy recovery from infections.

Chapter 47: Unveiling the Complex Relationship Between Cortisol and the Body's Response to Trauma

We will delve into the intricate relationship between cortisol and the body's response to trauma. Cortisol, commonly known as the "stress hormone," plays a vital role in our body's stress response and various physiological processes. Trauma refers to an overwhelming event that can have profound physical and psychological effects on an individual. In this chapter, we will explore how cortisol is intricately involved in the body's response to trauma, shedding light on the mechanisms at play and offering insights into understanding and managing trauma from a physiological perspective.

Understanding Cortisol and the Body's Response to Trauma:

Before we explore the specifics of cortisol's relationship with trauma, let's establish a foundational understanding of these terms. Cortisol is a hormone produced by the adrenal glands in response to stress. It helps regulate various physiological processes, including metabolism, immune function, blood pressure regulation, and inflammation. Trauma encompasses a range of experiences that involve physical harm, emotional distress, or psychological shock, such as accidents, violence, natural disasters, or witnessing or experiencing traumatic events.

Cortisol's Role in the Body's Response to Trauma:

Cortisol plays a significant role in the body's response to trauma through various mechanisms. Here's a closer look at how cortisol and trauma interact:

Activation of the Stress Response:

When an individual experiences trauma, the body's stress response is activated. This response involves the release of cortisol and other stress hormones, triggering a cascade of physiological changes. Cortisol helps mobilize energy reserves, heightens alertness, and readies the body for immediate action or protection in the face of danger.

Adaptive Stress Response:

The acute release of cortisol during and immediately after a traumatic event serves as an adaptive response. It enables the body to react quickly, promoting survival by enhancing focus, arousal, and physical readiness. Cortisol helps regulate blood pressure, blood sugar levels, and immune responses, preparing the body to cope with the immediate demands of the situation.

Memory Formation and Emotional Processing:

Cortisol influences memory formation and emotional processing, which are key components of the trauma response. While cortisol facilitates the consolidation of emotionally significant memories, it can also modulate memory retrieval and the emotional intensity associated with traumatic experiences. This complex interplay between cortisol and memory can contribute to both the persistence and alteration of traumatic memories.

Regulation of Inflammation:

Inflammation is a natural response to trauma, helping to heal injured tissues. Cortisol plays a role in regulating the inflammatory response, preventing excessive inflammation, and supporting the resolution of inflammation. By modulating the release of pro-inflammatory molecules, cortisol helps maintain a balanced inflammatory response following trauma.

Effects of Cortisol on Trauma Recovery:

Understanding the effects of cortisol on trauma recovery can provide insights into the body's response and potential implications for healing. Here are some key considerations:

Impact on Emotional Well-being:

Cortisol's influence on emotional processing can affect an individual's response to trauma and subsequent emotional well-being. Alterations in cortisol levels and dysregulation of the stress response may contribute to the development of post-traumatic stress disorder (PTSD) or other trauma-related mental health conditions. Managing stress and seeking appropriate therapeutic interventions can support emotional healing and resilience.

Healing and Inflammation:

Cortisol's anti-inflammatory properties can aid in the healing process following physical trauma. By controlling inflammation, cortisol helps reduce tissue damage and supports the repair and regeneration of injured tissues. However, excessive, or prolonged cortisol release can interfere with the normal healing process and potentially delay recovery.

Sleep Disturbances:

Trauma can disrupt sleep patterns, and cortisol dysregulation may contribute to sleep disturbances. Elevated cortisol levels at night can interfere with the natural sleep-wake cycle, leading to difficulties falling asleep, frequent awakenings, or nightmares. Creating a conducive sleep environment and implementing relaxation techniques can help promote restful sleep and support the body's healing processes.

Resilience and Coping:

Individual responses to trauma and cortisol release can vary significantly. Factors such as previous experiences, support systems, genetics, and overall resilience can influence an individual's ability to cope with and recover from traumatic events. Implementing healthy coping strategies, seeking professional support, and fostering a supportive environment are essential in facilitating resilience and healing.

So,

Cortisol, as a key hormone involved in the stress response, plays a complex role in the body's response to trauma. Understanding the interplay between cortisol and trauma provides insights into the physiological mechanisms at play and potential implications for trauma recovery.

By managing stress levels, seeking appropriate therapeutic interventions, prioritizing emotional well-being, ensuring adequate rest and sleep, and fostering a supportive environment, individuals can support their body's response to trauma. Remember, trauma recovery is a multifaceted process that may require professional guidance and support. With a comprehensive approach to healing, it is possible to navigate the path toward resilience and restoration following traumatic experiences.

Chapter 48: The Intricate Dance Between Cortisol and the Body's Response to Environmental Pollutants

We will explore the fascinating relationship between cortisol and the body's response to environmental pollutants. Cortisol, commonly known as the "stress hormone," plays a vital role in our body's stress response and various physiological processes. Environmental pollutants, such as air pollutants, heavy metals, pesticides, and other toxic substances, can have detrimental effects on human health. In this chapter, we will delve into the details of how cortisol impacts the body's response to environmental pollutants, shedding light on the mechanisms involved and offering insights into understanding and mitigating the potential health risks associated with exposure to pollutants.

Understanding Cortisol and Environmental Pollutants:

Before we dive into the specifics of cortisol's relationship with environmental pollutants, let's establish a foundational understanding of these terms. Cortisol is a hormone produced by the adrenal glands in response to stress. It helps regulate various physiological processes, including metabolism, immune function, blood pressure regulation, and inflammation. Environmental pollutants encompass a wide range of toxic substances present in the air, water, soil, and various consumer products that can have harmful effects on human health when exposed to them.

Cortisol's Impact on the Body's Response to Environmental Pollutants:

Cortisol can influence the body's response to environmental pollutants through various mechanisms. Here's a closer look at how cortisol and environmental pollutants interact:

Activation of the Stress Response:

Exposure to environmental pollutants can trigger a stress response in the body. This response involves the release of cortisol and other stress hormones, mobilizing resources to cope with the perceived threat. Cortisol helps regulate the physiological changes associated with stress, including the modulation of inflammation and immune responses.

Inflammatory Response:

Environmental pollutants, such as air pollutants and certain chemicals, can induce inflammation in the body. Cortisol has potent anti-inflammatory properties, which can help mitigate the inflammatory response triggered by exposure to pollutants. By modulating the release of pro-inflammatory molecules, cortisol plays a crucial role in dampening excessive inflammation and promoting the resolution of inflammatory processes.

Oxidative Stress:

Many environmental pollutants exert their toxic effects by promoting oxidative stress in the body. Oxidative stress occurs when there is an imbalance between the production of harmful reactive oxygen species (ROS) and the body's antioxidant defense mechanisms. Cortisol, as an anti-inflammatory and immunosuppressive hormone, can help regulate oxidative stress by reducing inflammation and modulating the immune response to oxidative damage.

Immune System Modulation:

Exposure to environmental pollutants can disrupt immune function and compromise the body's ability to defend against pathogens and toxins. Cortisol plays a role in modulating immune responses, including the suppression of certain aspects of immune function. While this immunosuppressive effect may be beneficial in mitigating excessive immune reactions, prolonged or excessive cortisol release can compromise immune defense mechanisms.

Effects of Cortisol on Health Risks Associated with Environmental Pollutants:

Understanding the effects of cortisol on health risks associated with environmental pollutants can provide insights into potential strategies for minimizing adverse outcomes. Here are some key considerations:

Individual Susceptibility:

The impact of cortisol on health risks associated with environmental pollutants can vary among individuals. Factors such as genetics, overall health status, lifestyle choices, and exposure levels can influence the body's response to pollutants and the interplay with cortisol. It is important to assess individual susceptibility and consider personalized approaches to minimize exposure and optimize health outcomes.

Stress Management:

Given that exposure to environmental pollutants can induce a stress response and cortisol release, effective stress management techniques are crucial. Engaging in stress reduction practices, such as mindfulness, exercise, relaxation techniques, and adequate sleep, can help mitigate the impact of stress on cortisol levels and support overall well-being in the face of environmental pollutant exposure.

Antioxidant Support:

As environmental pollutants often promote oxidative stress, supporting the body's antioxidant defense mechanisms becomes crucial. Consuming a diet rich in antioxidants, such as fruits, vegetables, and whole grains, can help counteract the harmful effects of pollutants. Additionally, lifestyle choices, such as avoiding smoking and reducing exposure to other environmental toxins, can further support antioxidant capacity.

Environmental Awareness and Protection:

Promoting awareness and taking measures to reduce exposure to environmental pollutants are essential for mitigating health risks. This includes advocating for clean air policies, practicing proper waste management, utilizing protective equipment in occupational settings, and making informed consumer choices regarding the use of household products and pesticides.

So,

Cortisol, as a key hormone involved in the stress response, can influence the body's response to environmental pollutants. Understanding the interplay between cortisol and environmental pollutants provides insights into potential strategies for minimizing health risks and optimizing well-being.

By managing stress levels, practicing effective stress reduction techniques, supporting antioxidant defenses, and advocating for environmental protection, individuals can minimize the potential adverse effects associated with exposure to environmental pollutants.

Remember, it is crucial to stay informed about environmental risks, prioritize health-conscious choices, and consult with healthcare professionals or environmental experts for guidance on minimizing exposure and optimizing health outcomes in the face of environmental pollutant exposure.

Chapter 49: Unraveling the Connection Between Cortisol and Chronic Pain Conditions

We will explore the intriguing relationship between cortisol and chronic pain conditions. Cortisol, commonly known as the "stress hormone," plays a crucial role in our body's stress response and various physiological processes. Chronic pain conditions, such as fibromyalgia, chronic back pain, arthritis, and neuropathic pain, can significantly impact an individual's quality of life. In this chapter, we will delve into the details of how cortisol may play a role in the development and progression of chronic pain conditions, shedding light on the mechanisms involved and offering insights into understanding and managing these complex pain disorders.

Understanding Cortisol and Chronic Pain Conditions:

Before we delve into the specifics of cortisol's relationship with chronic pain, let's establish a foundational understanding of these terms. Cortisol is a hormone produced by the adrenal glands in response to stress. It helps regulate various physiological processes, including metabolism, immune function, blood pressure regulation, and inflammation. Chronic pain conditions refer to persistent pain that lasts for extended periods, typically beyond the expected time for tissue healing.

Cortisol's Potential Role in Chronic Pain Conditions:

While the precise role of cortisol in chronic pain conditions is complex and multifactorial, research suggests several mechanisms through which cortisol may influence pain perception and the development and progression of chronic pain. Here's a closer look at how cortisol and chronic pain conditions interact:

Modulation of Inflammation:

Cortisol has potent anti-inflammatory properties that can help regulate inflammation, a common feature in many chronic pain conditions. Inflammatory processes can sensitize pain receptors, contributing to the amplification and persistence of pain signals. Cortisol's anti-inflammatory effects may help modulate these inflammatory responses, potentially providing some relief from chronic pain symptoms.

Pain Threshold and Sensitization:

Cortisol can influence pain sensitivity and the pain threshold, the point at which a stimulus is perceived as painful. Elevated cortisol levels have been associated with decreased pain sensitivity, while lower levels may contribute to increased pain perception. Cortisol can modulate pain signals in the central nervous system, influencing the transmission and interpretation of pain signals.

Stress and Pain Perception:

Chronic pain conditions are often associated with heightened stress levels, which can impact cortisol release. Stress-induced cortisol release may contribute to alterations in pain perception and pain modulation mechanisms. Chronic stress and dysregulation of the stress response can disrupt the delicate balance between cortisol and pain regulation, potentially exacerbating chronic pain symptoms.

Psychological Factors:

Psychological factors, such as anxiety, depression, and stress, commonly coexist with chronic pain conditions. These factors can influence cortisol levels and the body's response to pain. Higher cortisol levels have been associated with greater psychological distress, which can intensify pain experiences. Psychological interventions that target stress reduction and emotional well-being may help modulate cortisol levels and alleviate chronic pain symptoms.

Effects of Cortisol on Chronic Pain Management:

Understanding the effects of cortisol on chronic pain conditions can provide insights into potential strategies for managing these complex pain disorders. Here are some key considerations:

Stress Management:

Given the relationship between stress, cortisol, and chronic pain, effective stress management techniques are crucial. Stress reduction practices, such as mindfulness meditation, deep breathing exercises, relaxation techniques, and cognitive-behavioral therapy (CBT), can help modulate cortisol levels and reduce stress-related exacerbations of chronic pain symptoms.

Lifestyle Modifications:

Adopting a healthy lifestyle can positively influence cortisol levels and chronic pain management. Regular physical activity, proper nutrition, adequate sleep, and maintaining a balanced daily routine can support overall well-being and help mitigate the impact of cortisol dysregulation on chronic pain conditions.

Psychological Support:

Psychological interventions, such as CBT, mindfulness-based stress reduction, and relaxation therapies, can be beneficial for individuals with chronic pain. These approaches aim to enhance coping skills, reduce stress, and improve emotional well-being, potentially leading to improved pain management and cortisol regulation.

Medications and Interventions:

In some cases, healthcare professionals may recommend medications or interventions to manage chronic pain symptoms. These may include analgesic medications, anti-inflammatory drugs, physical therapy, acupuncture, or other specialized pain management techniques. It is important to work closely with healthcare providers to develop an individualized treatment plan that considers both the pain condition and cortisol regulation.

So,

The relationship between cortisol and chronic pain conditions is complex and multifaceted. While cortisol may play a role in the development and progression of chronic pain, it is important to recognize that pain is a complex phenomenon influenced by various factors, including physical, psychological, and environmental elements. By managing stress levels, adopting a healthy lifestyle, seeking psychological support, and collaborating with healthcare professionals to develop personalized treatment plans, individuals can optimize their management of chronic pain conditions. Remember, chronic pain is a multidimensional experience, and it may require a holistic approach that addresses physical, psychological, and social aspects of pain management. With comprehensive care and support, it is possible to enhance well-being and improve quality of life for individuals living with chronic pain.

Chapter 50: The Sun's Radiance: Exploring the Connection Between Cortisol, Sunlight, and Vitamin D

We will explore the fascinating relationship between cortisol, exposure to natural sunlight, and vitamin D levels. Cortisol, commonly known as the "stress hormone," plays a vital role in our body's stress response and various physiological processes. Natural sunlight, with its radiant warmth, brings us both physical and mental rejuvenation. Additionally, sunlight enables our bodies to produce vitamin D, a crucial nutrient for overall health. In this chapter, we will delve into the details of how cortisol levels may be influenced by exposure to natural sunlight and vitamin D, shedding light on the mechanisms involved and offering insights into the importance of embracing the sun's radiance for our well-being.

Understanding Cortisol, Sunlight, and Vitamin D:

Before we delve into the specifics of their relationship, let's establish a foundational understanding of cortisol, sunlight, and vitamin D. Cortisol is a hormone produced by the adrenal glands in response to stress. It helps regulate various physiological processes, including metabolism, immune function, blood pressure regulation, and inflammation. Sunlight, specifically the ultraviolet B (UVB) rays present in sunlight, stimulates our skin to produce vitamin D, a crucial nutrient involved in bone health, immune function, and other vital processes.

Cortisol's Relationship with Sunlight and Vitamin D:

Exposure to natural sunlight and the subsequent production of vitamin D can influence cortisol levels through various mechanisms. Here's a closer look at how cortisol, sunlight, and vitamin D interact:

Circadian Rhythm Regulation:

Exposure to natural sunlight helps regulate our circadian rhythm, the internal clock that governs various physiological processes, including the timing of cortisol release. Sunlight exposure in the morning helps synchronize our internal clock, promoting cortisol release in alignment with the natural daylight cycle. This synchronization helps optimize our energy levels, sleep patterns, and overall well-being.

Stress Reduction:

Natural sunlight and spending time outdoors in nature have been linked to stress reduction. Being in sunlight-rich environments can have a positive impact on our mood, promoting relaxation and reducing stress levels. As cortisol is intimately involved in the stress response, the stress-reducing effects of sunlight exposure can contribute to maintaining healthy cortisol levels.

Vitamin D and Cortisol Regulation:

Vitamin D plays a crucial role in modulating cortisol levels. Research suggests that optimal vitamin D levels can help regulate cortisol production and reduce excessive cortisol release. Adequate vitamin D levels may help prevent the dysregulation of the stress response and promote a balanced cortisol profile.

Immune System Function:

Both cortisol and vitamin D play critical roles in immune system function. Cortisol helps regulate immune responses, while vitamin D supports immune cell function and modulates the immune system. Adequate sunlight exposure and subsequent vitamin D production contribute to maintaining a healthy immune system, which can indirectly impact cortisol levels by promoting overall well-being.

Effects of Sunlight and Vitamin D on Cortisol Regulation:

Understanding the effects of sunlight exposure and vitamin D on cortisol regulation can provide insights into the importance of embracing the sun's radiance for our well-being. Here are some key considerations:

Optimal Sunlight Exposure:

Aiming for regular, moderate sunlight exposure can support cortisol regulation and overall health. It is important to strike a balance between enjoying the sun's benefits and avoiding excessive exposure that can lead to sunburn or other skin-related issues. The duration and intensity of sunlight exposure vary depending on factors such as geographical location, time of year, and individual skin type. Consulting guidelines or seeking advice from healthcare professionals can help determine the appropriate amount of sunlight exposure for each individual.

Vitamin D Supplementation:

In regions with limited sunlight exposure or for individuals with difficulty synthesizing vitamin D, supplementation may be necessary. Adequate vitamin D levels can support cortisol regulation and overall well-being. Consulting with healthcare professionals and getting regular blood tests can help determine whether vitamin D supplementation is needed and the appropriate dosage.

Mindful Sun Exposure:

While sunlight exposure is beneficial, it is important to practice sun safety measures. Applying sunscreen, wearing protective clothing, and seeking shade during peak sunlight hours can help prevent sunburn and reduce the risk of skin damage. Being mindful of sun exposure and taking necessary precautions can support long-term health benefits while minimizing potential risks.

Individual Variability:

The impact of sunlight exposure and vitamin D levels on cortisol regulation may vary among individuals. Factors such as skin type, geographical location, time spent outdoors, and overall health status can influence the body's response to sunlight and vitamin D. It is important to listen to your body, pay attention to any potential adverse effects, and consult with healthcare professionals for personalized guidance.

So,

The interplay between cortisol, natural sunlight, and vitamin D is a fascinating area of study. Embracing the sun's radiance and ensuring adequate vitamin D levels can contribute to maintaining healthy cortisol regulation and overall well-being.

By spending time outdoors, practicing sun safety measures, considering vitamin D supplementation when necessary, and seeking a balanced approach to sunlight exposure, individuals can harness the beneficial effects of sunlight while supporting optimal cortisol levels. Remember, each person's sun exposure needs may vary, and it is essential to find the right balance that works for you. Enjoy the sun's warm embrace and embrace the radiance it brings to your life.

Chapter 51: Cortisol's Role in the Body's Response to Surgical Procedures: A Journey Towards Healing

We will embark on a journey through the impact of cortisol on the body's response to surgical procedures. Cortisol, commonly known as the "stress hormone," plays a pivotal role in our body's stress response and various physiological processes. Surgical procedures, whether minor or major, are significant events that can cause stress and elicit complex physiological responses. In this chapter, we will explore the intricate relationship between cortisol and the body's response to surgery, shedding light on the mechanisms involved and offering insights into understanding and optimizing the healing process.

Understanding Cortisol and the Surgical Experience:

Before we dive into the specifics of cortisol's impact on surgery, let's establish a foundational understanding of cortisol and the surgical experience. Cortisol is a hormone produced by the adrenal glands in response to stress. It helps regulate various physiological processes, including metabolism, immune function, blood pressure regulation, and inflammation. Surgical procedures involve the intentional alteration of the body's tissues or organs to diagnose, treat, or repair certain medical conditions.

Cortisol's Impact on the Body's Response to Surgery:

Cortisol plays a significant role in the body's response to surgery through various mechanisms. Here's a closer look at how cortisol and surgical procedures interact:

Activation of the Stress Response:

Surgery, regardless of its nature, is perceived as a stressor by the body. As a result, the stress response is activated, leading to the release of cortisol and other stress hormones. Cortisol helps mobilize energy reserves, regulates blood pressure, and prepares the body for the physiological demands of surgery.

Inflammatory and Immune Responses:

Surgery triggers an inflammatory response as the body initiates healing processes and defends against potential infections. Cortisol, with its potent anti-inflammatory properties, helps regulate the inflammatory response, preventing excessive inflammation and promoting the resolution of the inflammatory process. By modulating the immune response, cortisol aids in minimizing the risk of postoperative complications.

Metabolic Effects:

Surgical procedures can have metabolic implications as the body adapts to the stress of surgery and the subsequent healing process. Cortisol influences metabolism by promoting the breakdown of stored nutrients, such as glycogen and fat, to provide energy for the body's needs. It also supports the production of glucose, the primary energy source during periods of stress.

Wound Healing and Tissue Repair:

Cortisol is involved in various aspects of wound healing and tissue repair. It helps regulate collagen synthesis, the formation of new blood vessels (angiogenesis), and the remodeling of tissues. Adequate cortisol levels are necessary for the proper progression of wound healing, promoting the closure of surgical incisions and the regeneration of damaged tissues.

Effects of Cortisol on Surgical Recovery and Healing:

Understanding the effects of cortisol on surgical recovery and healing can provide insights into optimizing the healing process. Here are some key considerations:

Stress Management:

Managing stress before and after surgery is essential for optimizing cortisol levels and overall well-being. Engaging in stress reduction techniques, such as deep breathing exercises, mindfulness meditation, gentle movement, and seeking emotional support, can help mitigate stress and support a more balanced cortisol response during the surgical journey.

Pain Management:

Surgery is often accompanied by pain, which can impact cortisol levels and overall recovery. Effective pain management strategies, such as appropriate medication regimens, physical therapy, and complementary therapies (e.g., acupuncture or relaxation techniques), can help reduce pain and minimize cortisol dysregulation, facilitating a smoother healing process.

Nutrition and Hydration:

Adequate nutrition and hydration are crucial for supporting the healing process and optimizing cortisol regulation. Consuming a balanced diet that includes sufficient protein, vitamins, and minerals supports tissue repair and immune function. Hydration is also essential for maintaining optimal blood flow and cellular processes. It is important to follow any dietary guidelines provided by healthcare professionals to promote proper healing.

Sleep and Rest:

Quality sleep and sufficient rest are vital for recovery after surgery. Cortisol levels follow a diurnal pattern, with lower levels at night to support restorative sleep. Prioritizing a sleep-friendly environment, practicing relaxation techniques before bed, and maintaining a regular sleep schedule can help optimize cortisol regulation and support the body's healing processes.

Follow-up Care and Rehabilitation:

Postoperative care and rehabilitation play a significant role in the recovery process. Adhering to healthcare professionals' recommendations regarding wound care, medication usage, physical therapy, and follow-up visits can help facilitate optimal healing and minimize complications. Rehabilitation programs tailored to individual needs aid in restoring physical function, improving strength, and promoting overall well-being.

So,

Cortisol, as a key hormone involved in the stress response, plays a vital role in the body's response to surgical procedures. Understanding the interplay between cortisol and surgery provides insights into the physiological processes at play and potential strategies for optimizing healing.

By managing stress, effectively managing pain, prioritizing nutrition, and hydration, ensuring adequate sleep and rest, and adhering to postoperative care and rehabilitation plans, individuals can support their body's healing journey after surgery. Remember, every surgical experience is unique, and it is important to communicate closely with healthcare professionals, follow their guidance, and seek support when needed. With comprehensive care, patience, and a positive mindset, individuals can navigate the path towards a successful surgical recovery and healing.

Chapter 52: The Intricate Dance Between Cortisol and the Body's Response to Psychological Therapies and Interventions

We will explore the fascinating relationship between cortisol and the body's response to psychological therapies and interventions. Cortisol, commonly known as the "stress hormone," plays a crucial role in our body's stress response and various physiological processes. Psychological therapies and interventions, such as psychotherapy, counseling, cognitive-behavioral therapy (CBT), and mindfulness practices, are powerful tools for promoting mental well-being and personal growth. In this chapter, we will delve into the details of how cortisol may impact the body's response to psychological therapies, shedding light on the mechanisms involved and offering insights into optimizing the therapeutic process.

Understanding Cortisol and Psychological Therapies:

Before we delve into the specifics of cortisol's impact on psychological therapies, let's establish a foundational understanding of cortisol and psychological interventions. Cortisol is a hormone produced by the adrenal glands in response to stress. It helps regulate various physiological processes, including metabolism, immune function, blood pressure regulation, and inflammation. Psychological therapies and interventions aim to promote emotional well-being, enhance coping skills, and alleviate psychological distress through various techniques and approaches.

Cortisol's Potential Influence on the Body's Response to Psychological Therapies:

Cortisol can influence the body's response to psychological therapies through various mechanisms. Here's a closer look at how cortisol and psychological interventions may interact:

Stress Reduction:

Psychological therapies and interventions often target stress reduction and emotional regulation. High levels of chronic stress can dysregulate cortisol production and contribute to psychological distress. Effective psychological interventions can help reduce stress levels, promote relaxation, and modulate the stress response, which can have a positive impact on cortisol regulation.

Emotional Processing and Regulation:

Cortisol can influence emotional processing and regulation, which are essential components of psychological therapies. It plays a role in memory consolidation, emotional memory retrieval, and the regulation of emotional responses. Psychological interventions can help individuals navigate and process emotions effectively, potentially influencing cortisol levels and facilitating emotional healing.

Neuroplasticity and Brain Function:

Cortisol is intricately involved in neuroplasticity, the brain's ability to change and reorganize itself. Psychological therapies and interventions can promote positive changes in brain structure and function. By modulating cortisol levels, these interventions can support neuroplasticity and facilitate the rewiring of neural pathways associated with adaptive behavior and emotional well-being.

Mindfulness and Cortisol Regulation:

Mindfulness practices, which involve paying attention to the present moment with non-judgmental awareness, have been shown to influence cortisol levels. Mindfulness-based interventions can reduce stress and lower cortisol levels, promoting a more balanced stress response. By cultivating mindfulness skills, individuals can enhance their ability to regulate emotions and respond to stressors, positively impacting the therapeutic process.

Effects of Cortisol on the Therapeutic Process:

Understanding the effects of cortisol on the therapeutic process can provide insights into optimizing psychological interventions. Here are some key considerations:

Therapeutic Alliance:

The therapeutic alliance, the relationship between the therapist and the client, is crucial for effective psychological interventions. High cortisol levels can impact interpersonal interactions and compromise the therapeutic alliance. It is important for therapists to create a supportive, non-judgmental environment that promotes trust and psychological safety, enabling clients to feel comfortable and engaged in the therapeutic process.

Stress Management Techniques:

Psychological interventions often include stress management techniques to help individuals cope with and reduce stress levels. By teaching stress reduction strategies, such as relaxation techniques, mindfulness practices, and cognitive restructuring, therapists can support individuals in modulating cortisol levels and improving overall well-being.

Emotional Regulation:

Cortisol's impact on emotional regulation underscores the importance of incorporating emotional regulation techniques in psychological therapies. Therapists can guide individuals in identifying and understanding their emotions, developing adaptive coping strategies, and fostering emotional resilience. By facilitating effective emotional regulation, therapists can help modulate cortisol responses and promote emotional well-being.

Timing of Interventions:

Considering the diurnal pattern of cortisol release is important when scheduling therapeutic interventions. Cortisol levels follow a circadian rhythm, with higher levels in the morning and lower levels in the evening. Planning sessions during times when cortisol levels are naturally lower may enhance the effectiveness of interventions and support the therapeutic process.

So,

Cortisol, as a key hormone involved in the stress response, can impact the body's response to psychological therapies and interventions. Understanding the interplay between cortisol and psychological interventions provides insights into optimizing the therapeutic process and promoting emotional well-being.

By addressing stress, incorporating stress management techniques, cultivating emotional regulation skills, and fostering a strong therapeutic alliance, psychologists and therapists can enhance the effectiveness of psychological interventions. Remember, each individual's response to therapy is unique, and it is important to tailor interventions to meet their specific needs. With compassionate guidance, evidence-based practices, and an understanding of cortisol's influence, psychological therapies can offer a pathway towards healing and personal growth.

Chapter 53: The Cortisol Connection: Unveiling the Role of Cortisol in Substance Abuse Disorders

We will delve into the intriguing relationship between cortisol and substance abuse disorders. Cortisol, commonly known as the "stress hormone," plays a crucial role in our body's stress response and various physiological processes. Substance abuse disorders, such as addiction to drugs or ..., have profound impacts on individuals and society. In this chapter, we will explore the complex interplay between cortisol and substance abuse, shedding light on the mechanisms involved and offering insights into understanding and addressing these challenging disorders.

Understanding Cortisol and Substance Abuse Disorders:

Before we delve into the specifics of cortisol's role in substance abuse disorders, let's establish a foundational understanding of cortisol and substance abuse. Cortisol is a hormone produced by the adrenal glands in response to stress. It helps regulate various physiological processes, including metabolism, immune function, blood pressure regulation, and inflammation. Substance abuse disorders refer to the chronic, compulsive misuse of substances, leading to negative consequences on physical, psychological, and social aspects of an individual's life.

Cortisol's Potential Influence on Substance Abuse Disorders:

Cortisol can potentially impact the development and progression of substance abuse disorders through various mechanisms. Here's a closer look at how cortisol and substance abuse interact:

Stress and Craving:

Stress is a significant factor in the development and maintenance of substance abuse disorders. Elevated cortisol levels are often associated with chronic stress. Stress-induced cortisol release can activate brain regions involved in reward and motivation, potentially increasing the likelihood of drug-seeking behavior and craving. The interplay between cortisol and the brain's reward system may contribute to the reinforcing effects of substances.

Self-Medication:

Individuals may turn to substance use as a way to self-medicate or cope with stress, anxiety, or other emotional distress. Cortisol dysregulation, often observed in individuals with chronic stress, can affect mood, motivation, and the body's stress response. Substance use may provide temporary relief by altering cortisol levels and influencing emotional states, leading to a cycle of self-medication and substance dependence.

Cortisol and Neuroadaptation:

Long-term substance abuse can lead to changes in the brain's structure and function, often referred to as neuroadaptation. Cortisol dysregulation can impact these neuroadaptations, potentially influencing the brain's response to substances. Chronic substance use can alter cortisol receptors in the brain, leading to changes in stress sensitivity and cortisol feedback mechanisms.

HPA Axis Dysregulation:

The hypothalamic-pituitary-adrenal (HPA) axis, which includes the release of cortisol, plays a crucial role in the body's stress response. Prolonged substance abuse can disrupt the HPA axis, leading to dysregulation of cortisol release. This dysregulation can further contribute to stress-related behaviors, craving, and potential relapse.

Effects of Cortisol on Substance Abuse Treatment and Recovery:

Understanding the effects of cortisol on substance abuse disorders can provide insights into optimizing treatment and recovery efforts. Here are some key considerations:

Stress Management Techniques:

Given the role of stress in substance abuse, stress management techniques are essential in treatment. Psychotherapy, counseling, mindfulness-based interventions, and stress reduction techniques can help individuals develop healthy coping mechanisms and reduce cortisol levels. By addressing stress, treatment can support long-term recovery and reduce the risk of relapse.

Medications and Cortisol Regulation:

Certain medications used in substance abuse treatment can influence cortisol levels. For example, medications such as naltrexone, used in the treatment of opioid and ... dependence, have been shown to modulate cortisol release. Healthcare professionals may consider medications that address both substance abuse and cortisol dysregulation to optimize treatment outcomes.

Comprehensive Care:

Comprehensive substance abuse treatment should address both the physical and psychological aspects of addiction. This includes providing support for stress management, emotional regulation, and overall well-being. Holistic approaches that incorporate nutritional support, physical activity, and mindfulness practices can contribute to cortisol regulation and enhance treatment efficacy.

Individualized Approach:

Every individual's experience with substance abuse and cortisol dysregulation is unique. Therefore, treatment plans should be individualized and tailored to address specific needs. A comprehensive assessment, including evaluation of stress levels and cortisol dysregulation, can guide the development of personalized treatment strategies.

So,

Cortisol, as a key hormone involved in the stress response, may play a role in the development and progression of substance abuse disorders. Understanding the interplay between cortisol and substance abuse provides insights into the complex mechanisms involved and potential strategies for intervention and recovery.

By addressing stress, incorporating stress management techniques, providing comprehensive care, and developing individualized treatment plans, professionals can optimize substance abuse treatment outcomes. It is crucial to consider the multifaceted nature of substance abuse disorders and the individual needs of each person on their path to recovery. With compassionate support, evidence-based interventions, and an understanding of cortisol's influence, we can move closer to helping individuals overcome substance abuse and embrace a healthier, more fulfilling life.

Chapter 54: Unraveling the Genetic Influence on Cortisol Levels: How Genes Shape the Stress Hormone

We will embark on a journey through the fascinating world of genetics and its influence on cortisol levels. Cortisol, commonly known as the "stress hormone," plays a pivotal role in our body's stress response and various physiological processes. Genetic factors, which contribute to the uniqueness of each individual, can impact cortisol regulation. In this chapter, we will explore the intricate relationship between genetics and cortisol levels, shedding light on the mechanisms involved and offering insights into understanding the genetic influence on this vital hormone.

Understanding Cortisol and Genetic Factors:

Before we dive into the specifics of genetic influence on cortisol levels, let's establish a foundational understanding of cortisol and genetic factors. Cortisol is a hormone produced by the adrenal glands in response to stress. It helps regulate various physiological processes, including metabolism, immune function, blood pressure regulation, and inflammation. Genetic factors refer to the inherited traits and variations in our DNA that contribute to individual differences.

Genetic Influence on Cortisol Levels:

Genetic factors can influence cortisol levels through various mechanisms. Here's a closer look at how genes shape the stress hormone:

Enzymes and Cortisol Metabolism:

Genetic variations in enzymes involved in cortisol metabolism can impact cortisol levels. For example, the enzyme 11β-HSD2 plays a role in converting cortisol to its inactive form, cortisone. Genetic variants in the gene encoding 11β-HSD2 can affect its activity, potentially leading to altered cortisol metabolism and levels.

Cortisol Receptors:

Genetic variations in cortisol receptors can influence their sensitivity and affinity for cortisol. The glucocorticoid receptor (GR), encoded by the NR3C1 gene, interacts with cortisol to regulate gene expression. Variations in the NR3C1 gene can affect the functioning of GR, potentially impacting cortisol feedback regulation and the body's response to stress.

Hypothalamic-Pituitary-Adrenal (HPA) Axis Genes:

Genetic variations in genes involved in the HPA axis, which regulates cortisol production, can impact cortisol levels. For example, variations in the genes encoding corticotropin-releasing hormone (CRH), adrenocorticotropic hormone (ACTH), and other HPA axis components can influence the HPA axis functioning and cortisol release.

Epigenetic Modifications:

Epigenetic modifications, which involve changes in gene expression without altering the DNA sequence, can impact cortisol regulation. Factors such as stress, environment, and lifestyle can influence epigenetic modifications, potentially affecting the expression of genes involved in cortisol metabolism and signaling pathways.

Effects of Genetic Influence on Cortisol Levels:

Understanding the effects of genetic factors on cortisol levels can provide insights into individual differences in stress responses and associated health outcomes. Here are some key considerations:

Stress Susceptibility:

Genetic variations related to cortisol regulation can influence an individual's susceptibility to stress. Some individuals may have genetic variations that result in higher or lower cortisol levels in response to stressors. This can contribute to differences in stress resilience and vulnerability to stress-related disorders.

Risk for Psychiatric Disorders:

Genetic factors influencing cortisol levels can impact an individual's susceptibility to psychiatric disorders. Dysregulation of cortisol has been implicated in conditions such as depression, anxiety disorders, and post-traumatic stress disorder (PTSD). Genetic variants that affect cortisol regulation may contribute to the risk and severity of these disorders.

Individual Stress Responses:

Genetic factors can shape an individual's stress response, influencing their physiological and psychological reactions to stress. Some individuals may be genetically predisposed to have a heightened or blunted cortisol response to stressors, impacting their ability to cope with and recover from stressful situations.

Treatment Response:

Genetic factors can also influence an individual's response to interventions targeting cortisol regulation. Understanding an individual's genetic profile may help personalize treatment approaches, optimizing therapeutic outcomes. For example, certain genetic variants may indicate a better response to specific medications or behavioral interventions.

So,

Genetic factors can influence cortisol levels, shaping an individual's stress response and associated health outcomes. Understanding the genetic influence on cortisol regulation provides insights into the complexity of individual stress responses and potential strategies for personalized interventions.

By considering genetic factors, healthcare professionals can tailor treatment approaches to better match an individual's genetic profile, optimizing therapeutic outcomes. However, it is important to recognize that genetic factors are just one piece of the puzzle, and they interact with environmental factors, lifestyle choices, and other influences. Emphasizing a holistic approach that takes into account both genetic and environmental factors can provide a more comprehensive understanding of cortisol regulation and its impact on health and well-being.

Ultimately, the interplay between genetics and cortisol levels highlights the uniqueness of each individual's stress response. By uncovering the genetic influence on cortisol, we gain a deeper understanding of our physiological differences and pave the way for personalized approaches to stress management and overall health.

Chapter 55: Cortisol and Acute Injuries:

Understanding the Body's Response to Recovery

We will explore the intriguing relationship between cortisol and the body's response to acute injuries. Cortisol, commonly known as the "stress hormone," plays a vital role in our body's stress response and various physiological processes. Acute injuries, such as fractures, sprains, or wounds, require a complex series of events for proper healing and recovery. In this chapter, we will delve into the details of how cortisol interacts with the body's response to acute injuries, shedding light on the mechanisms involved and offering insights into understanding the healing process.

Understanding Cortisol and Acute Injuries:

Before we dive into the specifics of cortisol's role in the body's response to acute injuries, let's establish a foundational understanding of cortisol and acute injuries. Cortisol is a hormone produced by the adrenal glands in response to stress. It helps regulate various physiological processes, including metabolism, immune function, blood pressure regulation, and inflammation. Acute injuries refer to sudden physical traumas that cause damage to tissues or structures within the body.

Cortisol's Impact on the Body's Response to Acute Injuries:

Cortisol can influence the body's response to acute injuries through various mechanisms. Here's a closer look at how cortisol interacts with the healing process:

Inflammation and Immune Response:

Following an acute injury, the body initiates an inflammatory response to remove damaged tissue and initiate healing. Cortisol, as a potent anti-inflammatory hormone, helps regulate the intensity and duration of the inflammatory response. It acts by suppressing the production of pro-inflammatory substances, thus reducing inflammation. This can aid in controlling excessive inflammation and preventing further tissue damage.

Pain Perception:

Acute injuries often lead to pain as a protective mechanism. Cortisol can modulate the perception of pain by influencing the transmission and processing of pain signals in the central nervous system. It can dampen pain signals, leading to pain relief and improved comfort during the recovery process.

Collagen Production and Tissue Repair:

Collagen, a protein crucial for tissue repair and wound healing, plays a vital role in the recovery from acute injuries. Cortisol can affect collagen synthesis by influencing the activity of fibroblasts, the cells responsible for producing collagen. Optimal cortisol levels are necessary to maintain the balance between collagen production and degradation, promoting proper tissue repair.

Energy Metabolism:

Acute injuries require energy for the healing process. Cortisol plays a role in regulating energy metabolism by mobilizing glucose, the body's primary energy source. It facilitates the breakdown of glycogen (stored glucose) and stimulates gluconeogenesis (the production of glucose from non-carbohydrate sources). This ensures that energy is available to support the repair and recovery processes.

Effects of Cortisol on Acute Injury Recovery:

Understanding the effects of cortisol on acute injury recovery can provide insights into optimizing the healing process. Here are some key considerations:

Stress Management:

The body's stress response, including cortisol release, can be activated by acute injuries. Managing stress levels is important to prevent excessive cortisol release, which may delay the healing process. Stress reduction techniques such as relaxation exercises, mindfulness practices, and social support can help modulate cortisol levels and promote optimal healing.

Nutritional Support:

Cortisol's influence on energy metabolism highlights the importance of providing adequate nutrition during the recovery period. A balanced diet rich in nutrients, particularly protein, vitamins, and minerals, supports collagen synthesis and tissue repair. Working with a healthcare professional or a registered dietitian can ensure optimal nutrition for enhanced recovery.

Pain Management:

Cortisol's role in pain perception underscores the significance of effective pain management during the recovery process. A comprehensive approach to pain management, including medication, physical therapy, and complementary therapies, can help alleviate pain and improve the individual's comfort and overall well-being.

Exercise and Rehabilitation:

Proper exercise and rehabilitation are crucial components of acute injury recovery. Cortisol levels can be influenced by exercise intensity and duration. Balancing the exercise regimen to avoid excessive cortisol release while promoting muscle strength, flexibility, and functional recovery is key. Working with a qualified healthcare professional or physical therapist can ensure a tailored and safe rehabilitation program.

So,

Cortisol, as a key hormone involved in the stress response, can impact the body's response to acute injuries. Understanding the interplay between cortisol and acute injury recovery provides insights into the healing process and potential strategies for optimizing recovery outcomes.

By managing stress levels, providing nutritional support, implementing effective pain management strategies, and tailoring exercise and rehabilitation programs, individuals can enhance the body's natural healing abilities and promote a successful recovery from acute injuries. Remember, each injury and recovery process are unique, and it is important to consult with healthcare professionals for personalized guidance and support. With a holistic approach that takes into account the role of cortisol, we can foster optimal healing, allowing individuals to regain their physical well-being and resume their daily activities.

Chapter 56: Navigating the Hormonal Journey: Cortisol's Influence on Pregnancy and Maternal Well-being

We will embark on a journey through the intricate relationship between cortisol and the body's response to hormonal changes during pregnancy. Cortisol, commonly known as the "stress hormone," plays a crucial role in our body's stress response and various physiological processes. Pregnancy is a transformative period characterized by significant hormonal changes that support the development of new life. In this chapter, we will explore the impact of cortisol on pregnancy, shedding light on the mechanisms involved and offering insights into understanding the dynamic interplay between cortisol and maternal well-being.

Understanding Cortisol and Hormonal Changes during Pregnancy:

Before we delve into the specifics of cortisol's role in the body's response to hormonal changes during pregnancy, let's establish a foundational understanding of cortisol and the hormonal journey of pregnancy. Cortisol is a hormone produced by the adrenal glands in response to stress. It helps regulate various physiological processes, including metabolism, immune function, blood pressure regulation, and inflammation. During pregnancy, the body experiences significant hormonal shifts, driven by the interaction of various hormones such as estrogen, progesterone, and human chorionic gonadotropin (hCG).

Cortisol's Impact on the Body's Response to Hormonal Changes during Pregnancy:

Cortisol can influence the body's response to hormonal changes during pregnancy through various mechanisms. Here's a closer look at how cortisol interacts with the hormonal journey of pregnancy:

Stress Regulation:

Pregnancy is a time of heightened emotional and physical changes, which can lead to increased stress levels. Cortisol plays a crucial role in stress regulation, helping the body respond to and cope with stressors. However, excessive, or chronic stress during pregnancy

225

can result in dysregulated cortisol levels, potentially affecting maternal well-being and the developing fetus.

Immune System Modulation:

During pregnancy, the immune system undergoes changes to protect both the mother and the developing fetus. Cortisol, as an immunomodulatory hormone, influences immune responses. It helps maintain immune tolerance by dampening certain immune reactions that could potentially harm the fetus. Cortisol's influence on immune function is vital in preventing the rejection of the fetus as a foreign entity.

Metabolic Regulation:

Pregnancy requires significant metabolic adaptations to support the growing fetus. Cortisol is involved in regulating metabolism, including glucose metabolism and insulin sensitivity. It aids in ensuring adequate energy supply for both the mother and the developing fetus. However, excessive cortisol levels, such as those associated with chronic stress, can disrupt metabolic regulation, and potentially contribute to gestational diabetes or other metabolic disorders.

Fetal Development:

Cortisol can cross the placental barrier and influence fetal development. The developing fetus has its own cortisol production, which is essential for maturation of certain organs and tissues. However, dysregulation of maternal cortisol levels, such as in cases of chronic stress, can impact fetal cortisol production and potentially affect fetal growth and development.

Effects of Cortisol on Maternal Well-being during Pregnancy:
Understanding the effects of cortisol on maternal well-being during pregnancy can provide insights into optimizing the prenatal experience. Here are some key considerations:

Stress Management:

Managing stress levels during pregnancy is crucial for maternal well-being. Chronic or excessive stress can result in dysregulated cortisol levels, potentially impacting both maternal health and fetal development. Implementing stress management techniques such as relaxation exercises, mindfulness practices, and social support can help modulate cortisol levels and promote overall well-being.

Healthy Lifestyle Choices:

Maintaining a healthy lifestyle is important for managing cortisol levels during pregnancy. Adequate sleep, regular physical activity, and a balanced diet can support hormonal balance and stress regulation. Engaging in activities that promote relaxation and self-care can also help alleviate stress and promote a positive prenatal experience.

Prenatal Care and Support:

Regular prenatal care is essential for monitoring maternal health and ensuring optimal fetal development. Healthcare professionals can assess cortisol levels when necessary and provide guidance and support to manage stress and promote well-being during pregnancy. Open communication and a trusting relationship with healthcare providers can foster a supportive environment for the mother's physical and emotional health.

Emotional Well-being:

Cortisol's influence on mood and emotional well-being underscores the importance of addressing mental health during pregnancy. Pregnancy can bring about a range of emotions, and it is crucial to prioritize emotional well-being. Engaging in activities that promote relaxation, seeking emotional support, and considering therapy or counseling can contribute to a positive emotional state during this transformative time.

So,

Cortisol, as a key hormone involved in the stress response, can impact the body's response to hormonal changes during pregnancy. Understanding the interplay between cortisol and the hormonal journey of pregnancy provides insights into optimizing maternal well-being and promoting a positive prenatal experience.

By managing stress levels, adopting a healthy lifestyle, seeking prenatal care and support, and prioritizing emotional well-being, mothers can navigate the hormonal changes of pregnancy with greater ease. Remember, each pregnancy is unique, and it is important to consult with healthcare professionals for personalized guidance and support.

With a holistic approach that considers the impact of cortisol, we can foster a nurturing environment for both the mother and the developing fetus, promoting a healthy and positive pregnancy experience.

Chapter 57: Unraveling the Complex Connection: Cortisol's Role in Eating Disorders

We will explore the intricate relationship between cortisol and the development and progression of eating disorders. Cortisol, commonly known as the "stress hormone," plays a vital role in our body's stress response and various physiological processes. Eating disorders, such as anorexia nervosa, bulimia nervosa, and binge eating disorder, are complex mental health conditions characterized by disturbances in eating behaviors and a distorted perception of body weight and shape. In this chapter, we will delve into the details of how cortisol interacts with eating disorders, shedding light on the mechanisms involved and offering insights into understanding the complex interplay between cortisol and these debilitating conditions.

Understanding Cortisol and Eating Disorders:

Before we delve into the specifics of cortisol's role in the development and progression of eating disorders, let's establish a foundational understanding of cortisol and eating disorders. Cortisol is a hormone produced by the adrenal glands in response to stress. It helps regulate various physiological processes, including metabolism, immune function, blood pressure regulation, and inflammation. Eating disorders are multifaceted conditions that involve psychological, genetic, environmental, and sociocultural factors.

Cortisol's Influence on Eating Disorders:

Cortisol can influence the development and progression of eating disorders through various mechanisms. Here's a closer look at how cortisol interacts with these complex conditions:

Stress Response and Emotional Regulation:

Eating disorders often coexist with high levels of chronic stress and emotional dysregulation. Cortisol, as a key stress hormone, is involved in the body's response to stress and can impact emotional regulation. Excessive or dysregulated cortisol levels, which can occur due to chronic stress, may contribute to emotional disturbances commonly associated with eating disorders, such as anxiety and depression.

Metabolism and Energy Balance:

Cortisol plays a role in regulating metabolism and energy balance. It can influence appetite, food intake, and the breakdown of macronutrients. Dysregulation of cortisol levels, such as in cases of chronic stress, may disrupt appetite regulation, leading to changes in eating behaviors and patterns. This can contribute to the development or maintenance of disordered eating behaviors seen in eating disorders.

Body Image and Body Dissatisfaction:

Distorted body image and dissatisfaction with body shape and weight are common features of eating disorders. Cortisol's impact on body composition and fat distribution may contribute to body dissatisfaction. Chronic stress and dysregulated cortisol levels can also contribute to body image concerns by influencing the release of other hormones involved in appetite regulation and body composition, such as leptin and ghrelin.

Neuroendocrine Dysregulation:

Cortisol interacts with various neuroendocrine systems involved in appetite regulation, reward processing, and mood regulation. Dysregulation of these systems, influenced by cortisol, can contribute to altered food reward processing, heightened food cravings, and difficulties in regulating food intake. These factors can exacerbate disordered eating behaviors and perpetuate the cycle of eating disorders.

Effects of Cortisol on Eating Disorders:

Understanding the effects of cortisol on eating disorders can provide insights into potential strategies for intervention and support. Here are some key considerations:

Stress Management:

Given the influence of cortisol on stress response and emotional regulation, stress management techniques are crucial in the treatment of eating disorders. Incorporating stress reduction strategies, such as mindfulness practices, relaxation exercises, and therapy focused on emotion regulation, can help modulate cortisol levels and support overall well-being.

Nutritional Rehabilitation:

Addressing nutritional needs is a key aspect of treating eating disorders. Cortisol's influence on appetite and metabolism highlights the importance of developing a balanced and structured meal plan. Working with registered dietitians who specialize in eating disorders can help individuals establish a nourishing relationship with food while considering cortisol's impact on metabolism.

Psychological Support:

Psychological interventions play a central role in treating eating disorders. Therapies such as cognitive-behavioral therapy (CBT), dialectical behavior therapy (DBT), and family-based therapy (FBT) can address the emotional and behavioral aspects of eating disorders. By targeting underlying psychological factors and promoting adaptive coping strategies, these therapies may indirectly impact cortisol levels and help individuals develop healthier relationships with food and their bodies.

Holistic Approach:

Recognizing the multifaceted nature of eating disorders, a holistic approach that considers various factors is essential. This includes addressing underlying psychological factors, working on stress management techniques, promoting self-compassion and body acceptance, and fostering a supportive environment that focuses on overall well-being rather than solely on weight or appearance.

So,

Cortisol, as a key hormone involved in the stress response, can influence the development and progression of eating disorders. Understanding the interplay between cortisol and eating disorders provides insights into the complex nature of these conditions and potential strategies for intervention and support.

By incorporating stress management techniques, addressing nutritional needs, providing psychological support, and adopting a holistic approach, healthcare professionals and support networks can help individuals on their journey toward recovery from eating disorders. It is crucial to approach treatment with empathy, understanding, and a focus on overall well-being, recognizing that recovery is a multifaceted process that may require ongoing support and personalized care.

Chapter 58: Unraveling the Electromagnetic Connection: Exploring the Influence of Electromagnetic Fields on Cortisol Levels

We embark on an exploration of the fascinating relationship between electromagnetic fields (EMFs) and cortisol levels. Cortisol, commonly known as the "stress hormone," plays a crucial role in our body's stress response and various physiological processes. EMFs, generated by various electrical and electronic devices, surround us in our modern technological world. In this chapter, we will delve into the details of how EMFs may influence cortisol levels, shedding light on the mechanisms involved and offering insights into understanding the potential impact of EMFs on our well-being.

Understanding Cortisol and Electromagnetic Fields:

Before we dive into the specifics of how EMFs may influence cortisol levels, let's establish a foundational understanding of cortisol and the nature of electromagnetic fields. Cortisol is a hormone produced by the adrenal glands in response to stress. It helps regulate various physiological processes, including metabolism, immune function, blood pressure regulation, and inflammation. Electromagnetic fields, on the other hand, refer to the invisible energy fields generated by the flow of electrical currents and the operation of electrical devices.

The Influence of Electromagnetic Fields on Cortisol Levels:

While the relationship between EMFs and cortisol levels is an area of ongoing research, several studies have explored the potential impact of EMFs on cortisol regulation. Here's a closer look at some key findings and considerations:

Stress Response:

Exposure to EMFs has been associated with alterations in the stress response system, including cortisol levels. Some studies suggest that exposure to high-frequency EMFs, such as those emitted by mobile phones or Wi-Fi networks, may increase cortisol levels, potentially indicating an activation of the stress response. However, the existing evidence is mixed, and further research is needed to establish a clear link between EMFs and cortisol response.

Sleep Disturbances:

Disruptions in sleep patterns can impact cortisol levels. EMF exposure, particularly from electronic devices used before sleep, has been found to affect sleep quality and duration. Poor sleep quality can contribute to increased cortisol levels and disrupt the natural cortisol rhythm. Limiting exposure to EMFs before bedtime, such as by avoiding screen time or using blue-light filters, may help promote better sleep and cortisol regulation.

Psychological Factors:

Psychological stress can influence cortisol levels, and some individuals may experience stress or anxiety related to EMF exposure. This psychological response to EMFs, known as electromagnetic hypersensitivity, can lead to physiological changes, including potential alterations in cortisol levels. However, it is important to note that electromagnetic hypersensitivity is not widely recognized as a medical diagnosis, and further research is needed to fully understand its impact on cortisol regulation.

Individual Variations:

Individual responses to EMFs and cortisol regulation can vary. Factors such as genetic predisposition, overall health status, and personal sensitivity may influence how individuals react to EMF exposure. Some people may be more susceptible to cortisol changes in response to EMFs, while others may show minimal or no noticeable effects. It is crucial to consider individual differences and experiences when exploring the relationship between EMFs and cortisol.

Mitigating the Potential Effects of Electromagnetic Fields:

While the scientific understanding of the relationship between EMFs and cortisol is still evolving, here are some practical considerations to mitigate potential effects:

Awareness and Mindful Usage:

Be mindful of your exposure to EMFs and consider ways to minimize unnecessary exposure. For example, keep electronic devices at a distance when not in use, use speakerphone or wired headsets instead of holding your phone close to your head, and take breaks from screens to reduce overall EMF exposure.

Sleep Hygiene:

Create a sleep-friendly environment by limiting exposure to electronic devices before bedtime. Establish a relaxing pre-sleep routine that does not involve screen time. Consider using blue-light filters on electronic devices or using devices specifically designed to reduce EMF emissions in the bedroom.

Personal Sensitivity:

If you feel that you may be particularly sensitive to EMFs or experience symptoms of electromagnetic hypersensitivity, consult with a healthcare professional who specializes in environmental sensitivities. They can provide guidance and support tailored to your individual needs.

Balanced Lifestyle:

Maintaining a healthy lifestyle that includes stress management techniques, regular exercise, adequate sleep, and a balanced diet can support overall well-being and potentially mitigate the impact of environmental factors, including EMFs, on cortisol regulation.

So,

The relationship between EMFs and cortisol levels is an area of ongoing research, and our understanding is still evolving. While some studies suggest a potential influence of EMFs on cortisol regulation, further research is needed to establish clear causal links and to determine individual variability in response.

In the meantime, being mindful of your exposure to EMFs, especially before bedtime, and adopting a balanced lifestyle that promotes overall well-being can help mitigate potential effects. It is important to stay informed about emerging research and consult with healthcare professionals for personalized guidance and support.

Remember, maintaining a healthy lifestyle and managing stress levels play vital roles in supporting optimal cortisol regulation and overall well-being. By staying proactive and informed, we can navigate the modern technological landscape while prioritizing our health and finding a balance that works best for us.

Type This URL in Your Browser → **https://bit.ly/Unbox_Your_SLIMCRYSTAL**

Chapter 59: Embracing the Elements: Cortisol's Influence on the Body's Response to Heat and Cold Stress

We explore the intriguing impact of cortisol on the body's response to heat and cold stress. Cortisol, known as the "stress hormone," plays a vital role in our body's stress response and various physiological processes. Our bodies have remarkable mechanisms to adapt to extreme temperatures, whether it's the scorching heat of a summer day or the bone-chilling cold of winter. In this chapter, we will delve into the details of how cortisol interacts with the body's response to heat and cold stress, shedding light on the mechanisms involved and offering insights into understanding the intricate interplay between cortisol and our thermal environment.

Understanding Cortisol and Heat/Cold Stress:

Before we delve into the specifics of cortisol's impact on the body's response to heat and cold stress, let's establish a foundational understanding of cortisol and how our bodies cope with extreme temperatures. Cortisol is a hormone produced by the adrenal glands in response to stress. It helps regulate various physiological processes, including metabolism, immune function, blood pressure regulation, and inflammation. When exposed to extreme heat or cold, our bodies activate intricate thermoregulatory mechanisms to maintain internal temperature homeostasis.

Cortisol's Influence on the Body's Response to Heat Stress:

When faced with heat stress, cortisol plays a multifaceted role in supporting the body's response. Here's a closer look at some key aspects:

Heat Perception and Thermoregulation:

Cortisol can influence the perception and regulation of body temperature. It interacts with various regions of the brain involved in temperature regulation, such as the hypothalamus, which plays a crucial role in maintaining thermal balance. Cortisol helps activate the heat dissipation mechanisms of the body, such as vasodilation (widening of blood vessels) and sweating, to facilitate heat loss and prevent overheating.

Inflammatory Response and Heat-Induced Stress:

Exposure to excessive heat can lead to heat-induced stress and inflammation. Cortisol, as an anti-inflammatory hormone, helps modulate the inflammatory response. It aids in minimizing excessive inflammation and the potential tissue damage associated with heat stress. By dampening the inflammatory response, cortisol contributes to maintaining tissue integrity and overall well-being during heat exposure.

Fluid and Electrolyte Balance:

Sweating is a crucial mechanism for dissipating heat from the body during hot conditions. Cortisol plays a role in fluid and electrolyte balance by regulating the reabsorption of sodium in the kidneys. This helps maintain appropriate electrolyte levels and supports the body's ability to maintain fluid balance during heat stress.

Cortisol's Influence on the Body's Response to Cold Stress:

In the face of cold stress, cortisol also plays a significant role in supporting the body's adaptive response. Here's an overview of its impact:

Cold Perception and Thermogenesis:

Cortisol influences the perception of cold and promotes thermogenesis, the production of heat by the body. It does so by stimulating the breakdown of stored energy sources, such as glycogen and fat, to generate heat. This process helps maintain body temperature and counteract the cold stress experienced.

Immune Function and Cold-Induced Stress:

Exposure to cold stress can temporarily suppress the immune system, making individuals more susceptible to infections. Cortisol, as an immunomodulatory hormone, can influence immune function during cold stress. It helps regulate immune responses, promoting a balanced and appropriate immune reaction to protect against potential pathogens.

Metabolic Adaptations:

Cold stress triggers metabolic adaptations aimed at generating heat. Cortisol is involved in these adaptations by promoting the breakdown of stored energy sources and increasing metabolic rate. These processes provide the necessary energy and heat production to help the body maintain thermal balance in cold environments.

Strategies for Supporting the Body's Response to Heat and Cold Stress: To optimize the body's response to heat and cold stress, here are some practical considerations:

Heat Stress:

• Stay hydrated by drinking plenty of water and electrolyte-rich fluids.
• Seek shade or air-conditioned environments during the hottest parts of the day.
• Wear lightweight, breathable clothing and use appropriate sun protection.
• Take regular breaks and rest in a cool environment when engaging in physical activities in high temperatures.

Cold Stress:

• Dress in layers to trap body heat and allow for adjustments based on temperature changes.
• Protect extremities by wearing warm socks, gloves, and hats.
• Seek shelter or warm environments during extreme cold weather conditions.
• Stay well-nourished to provide the body with energy for thermogenesis and heat production.

So,

Cortisol, as a key hormone involved in the stress response, influences the body's response to heat and cold stress. By understanding cortisol's impact on thermoregulation, inflammation, immune function, and metabolism, we can gain insights into optimizing our response to extreme temperatures.

Embracing the elements requires a balanced approach that considers individual needs and environmental conditions. By adopting strategies to support the body's thermoregulatory mechanisms, staying well-hydrated, dressing appropriately, and seeking shelter, when necessary, we can navigate the challenges of heat and cold stress while promoting our overall well-being.

Remember, it is important to listen to your body, respect its limits, and seek medical attention if you experience severe heat- or cold-related symptoms. Through a mindful approach to our thermal environment, we can adapt and thrive in the face of heat and cold stress, allowing us to embrace the beauty and diversity of our ever-changing world.

Chapter 60: Navigating the Medication Maze: Cortisol's Influence on the Body's Response and Drug Interactions

We explore the intricate relationship between cortisol and the body's response to medications and drug interactions. Cortisol, known as the "stress hormone," plays a vital role in our body's stress response and various physiological processes. When we take medications, it's important to understand how cortisol may impact their effectiveness and potential interactions. In this chapter, we will delve into the details of how cortisol interacts with medications, shedding light on the mechanisms involved and offering insights into understanding the potential influence of cortisol on our medication journeys.

Understanding Cortisol's Impact on Medication Response:

Before we delve into the specifics of cortisol's influence on medication response and drug interactions, let's establish a foundational understanding of cortisol and its role in our body. Cortisol is a hormone produced by the adrenal glands in response to stress. It helps regulate various physiological processes, including metabolism, immune function, blood pressure regulation, and inflammation. When it comes to medications, cortisol can affect their absorption, distribution, metabolism, and excretion—collectively known as pharmacokinetics—and their interactions with target receptors or enzymes—known as pharmacodynamics.

Cortisol's Influence on Pharmacokinetics:

Cortisol can influence the way medications are processed in our bodies. Here are some key considerations:

Absorption:

Cortisol's impact on the gastrointestinal tract and blood flow may affect the absorption of medications taken orally. Changes in cortisol levels can alter the rate and extent of drug absorption, potentially affecting their bioavailability and therapeutic effects.

Distribution:

Cortisol can influence the binding of medications to proteins in the blood, such as albumin. Changes in cortisol levels may affect the availability of these binding sites, which can alter the distribution of medications throughout the body. This can impact the effective concentration of drugs at their intended target sites.

Metabolism:

Cortisol interacts with various enzymes involved in drug metabolism, such as cytochrome P450 enzymes. Changes in cortisol levels can modulate the activity of these enzymes, potentially affecting the rate at which medications are metabolized. This, in turn, may impact their efficacy and safety profiles.

Excretion:

Cortisol can influence the excretion of medications from the body through its effects on renal function and urine production. Changes in cortisol levels may alter the elimination half-life of drugs, which can affect their duration of action and potential accumulation in the body.

Cortisol's Influence on Pharmacodynamics:

Beyond pharmacokinetics, cortisol can also impact the pharmacodynamics of medications. Here are some key considerations:

Receptor Interactions:

Cortisol can interact with receptors targeted by medications, potentially modulating their binding affinity or activation. This interaction can affect the effectiveness of medications and their ability to produce the desired therapeutic effects.

Enzyme Interactions:

Cortisol's influence on enzymes involved in drug metabolism can impact the conversion of medications to their active or inactive forms. This can influence the rate and extent of medication action and may contribute to interindividual variability in drug response.

Immune Function:

Cortisol, as an immunomodulatory hormone, can influence the immune response. Some medications rely on immune pathways to exert their therapeutic effects. Changes in cortisol levels can potentially impact the immune response, affecting the efficacy of these medications.

Navigating Medication Use and Interactions:
To optimize the use of medications and minimize potential interactions with cortisol, consider the following strategies:

Communication with Healthcare Providers:

Maintain open and honest communication with your healthcare providers regarding your medications, medical history, and any changes in your cortisol levels. This information can help guide medication selection, dosing adjustments, and potential modifications to your treatment plan.

Adherence to Prescribed Medication Regimens:

Follow the prescribed medication regimen as instructed by your healthcare provider. Consistency and adherence are key to achieving optimal therapeutic outcomes and reducing the potential for medication interactions.

Monitoring and Reporting:

Be aware of any changes in your symptoms, medication response, or side effects. If you experience any unusual or unexpected reactions, promptly report them to your healthcare provider. Regular monitoring of cortisol levels and medication efficacy can aid in identifying potential interactions or the need for dosage adjustments.

Lifestyle Factors:

Maintain a healthy lifestyle that includes proper nutrition, regular exercise, stress management techniques, and adequate sleep. These factors can contribute to overall well-being and may indirectly impact cortisol levels and medication response.
So,
Cortisol, as a key hormone involved in the stress response, can influence the body's response to medications and potential drug interactions. By understanding cortisol's impact on pharmacokinetics and pharmacodynamics, as well as implementing effective communication, adherence to medication regimens, monitoring, and a healthy lifestyle, we can navigate the medication maze with confidence. Remember, it is essential to consult with your healthcare provider regarding any concerns or questions about your medications. They can provide personalized guidance based on your specific health needs and medication regimen. By working together and staying informed, we can

optimize the benefits of medications while minimizing the potential for interactions with cortisol, ultimately supporting our overall health and well-being.

Chapter 61: Breathing Under the Influence: Exploring Cortisol's Impact on the Development and Progression of Lung Diseases

We dive into the intriguing relationship between cortisol and lung diseases. Cortisol, commonly known as the "stress hormone," plays a vital role in our body's stress response and various physiological processes. While its primary function is to help regulate stress, cortisol can also exert influences on immune function, inflammation, and tissue repair. In this chapter, we will explore the intricate interplay between cortisol and lung diseases, shedding light on how cortisol may contribute to the development and progression of respiratory conditions, and offering insights into potential mechanisms and therapeutic implications.

Understanding Cortisol's Influence on Lung Health:

Before we delve into the specifics of cortisol's impact on lung diseases, let's establish a foundational understanding of cortisol and the respiratory system. Cortisol is a hormone produced by the adrenal glands in response to stress. It helps regulate various physiological processes, including metabolism, immune function, and inflammation. The respiratory system comprises the airways, lungs, and associated structures involved in breathing and oxygen exchange.

Cortisol and Lung Diseases:

Emerging evidence suggests that cortisol may play a role in the development and progression of various lung diseases. Here's a closer look at some key respiratory conditions and the potential involvement of cortisol:

Asthma:

Asthma is a chronic inflammatory disease characterized by recurrent episodes of wheezing, breathlessness, chest tightness, and coughing. Cortisol has anti-inflammatory properties and plays a role in modulating immune responses. In asthma, dysregulation of cortisol and its receptors may contribute to airway inflammation and hyperresponsiveness. Imbalances in cortisol levels and impaired cortisol signaling may impact the severity and control of asthma symptoms.

Chronic Obstructive Pulmonary Disease (COPD):

COPD is a progressive lung disease characterized by airflow limitation and persistent respiratory symptoms. Cortisol dysregulation may contribute to the pathogenesis of COPD through its effects on inflammation, oxidative stress, and tissue remodeling. In COPD patients, altered cortisol levels and impaired glucocorticoid receptor signaling have been observed, which can impact the effectiveness of corticosteroid therapies.

Idiopathic Pulmonary Fibrosis (IPF):

IPF is a chronic and progressive interstitial lung disease characterized by the scarring and fibrosis of lung tissue. Cortisol has been implicated in the fibrotic process through its effects on immune regulation and tissue repair. Dysregulation of cortisol and impaired glucocorticoid signaling may contribute to the aberrant wound healing response in IPF, potentially influencing disease progression.

Respiratory Infections:

Respiratory infections, such as viral or bacterial infections, can trigger an immune response and inflammation in the airways. Cortisol, as an immunomodulatory hormone, plays a role in regulating the immune response to infection. Dysregulation of cortisol levels or impaired cortisol signaling may impact the body's ability to mount an appropriate immune response, potentially influencing the severity and duration of respiratory infections.

Mechanisms and Therapeutic Implications:

The mechanisms underlying cortisol's influence on lung diseases are complex and multifaceted. Here are some potential mechanisms and therapeutic implications:

Inflammation and Immune Regulation:

Cortisol exerts anti-inflammatory effects by suppressing immune responses and modulating the activity of immune cells. Dysregulation of cortisol levels or impaired cortisol signaling can lead to unresolved inflammation and abnormal immune responses, potentially contributing to lung disease pathogenesis. Targeting cortisol signaling pathways or using glucocorticoid therapies may offer therapeutic avenues for modulating inflammation in respiratory conditions.

Oxidative Stress and Antioxidant Defense:

Cortisol can influence oxidative stress, a condition characterized by an imbalance between the production of reactive oxygen species and the body's antioxidant defenses. Oxidative stress plays a role in lung injury and disease progression. Maintaining a balance in cortisol levels and optimizing antioxidant defense mechanisms may help mitigate oxidative stress-related damage in the lungs.

Tissue Repair and Remodeling:

Cortisol is involved in tissue repair and remodeling processes. In lung diseases characterized by fibrosis or tissue damage, dysregulation of cortisol and impaired glucocorticoid signaling can impact the repair mechanisms, potentially influencing disease progression. Strategies aimed at enhancing cortisol signaling or targeting specific signaling pathways involved in tissue repair may offer therapeutic potential.

Individual Variations and Personalized Medicine:

Individual differences in cortisol levels, sensitivity, and receptor expression may contribute to the variability in disease progression and treatment response among individuals with lung diseases. Understanding these individual variations and incorporating personalized medicine approaches may help optimize treatment strategies and improve patient outcomes.

So,

Cortisol's influence on lung diseases is an area of ongoing research, and our understanding continues to evolve. The intricate interplay between cortisol, immune function, inflammation, and tissue repair underscores its potential role in respiratory conditions. By unraveling the underlying mechanisms and considering personalized approaches, we can pave the way for new therapeutic strategies and enhance our ability to manage and treat lung diseases.

It is important to note that the management of respiratory conditions requires a comprehensive approach under the guidance of healthcare professionals. By staying informed, engaging in open communication with your healthcare provider, and following recommended treatment plans, you can work collaboratively to optimize your lung health and overall well-being. Through ongoing research and advancements in our understanding of cortisol's impact on lung diseases, we can strive for improved respiratory health for all.

Chapter 62: The Social Hormone: Exploring the Influence of Social Interactions and Support Networks on Cortisol Levels

We delve into the fascinating connection between cortisol levels and social interactions and support networks. Cortisol, commonly known as the "stress hormone," plays a vital role in our body's stress response and various physiological processes. While cortisol is primarily associated with stress, recent research has shed light on its relationship with our social lives. In this chapter, we will explore the intricate interplay between cortisol and social interactions, shedding light on how our social connections and support networks can influence cortisol levels, and offering insights into the potential implications for our well-being and overall health.

Understanding Cortisol and its Role in Stress:

Before we explore the influence of social interactions on cortisol levels, let's establish a foundational understanding of cortisol and stress. Cortisol is a hormone produced by the adrenal glands in response to stress. It helps regulate various physiological processes, including metabolism, immune function, and inflammation. When we encounter stressful situations, cortisol is released into our bloodstream, preparing our bodies for a "fight or flight" response.

The Influence of Social Interactions on Cortisol Levels:

Numerous studies have highlighted the impact of social interactions and support networks on cortisol levels. Here's a closer look at some key findings:

Social Support and Cortisol Regulation:

Strong social support networks have been linked to lower cortisol levels. Positive social interactions and supportive relationships can act as buffers against stress, reducing the release of cortisol. People with robust social connections tend to experience less physiological reactivity to stressful events and exhibit lower cortisol levels compared to those who are socially isolated.

Loneliness and Cortisol Dysregulation:

Conversely, feelings of loneliness and social isolation have been associated with dysregulated cortisol levels. Individuals who experience chronic loneliness may exhibit heightened cortisol reactivity, with higher baseline cortisol levels and greater cortisol release in response to stress. Prolonged loneliness can lead to a state of chronic stress, contributing to cortisol dysregulation.

Social Hierarchies and Cortisol:

Social hierarchies, such as those found in workplaces or social groups, can also influence cortisol levels. In competitive or hierarchical environments, individuals lower in the hierarchy may experience higher cortisol levels due to increased stress and perceived social threats. On the other hand, individuals higher in the hierarchy may exhibit lower cortisol levels, reflecting a sense of security and reduced stress.

Positive Social Interactions and Cortisol Reduction:

Engaging in positive social interactions, such as laughter, supportive conversations, and physical touch, has been associated with reduced cortisol levels. These interactions trigger the release of oxytocin, a hormone associated with bonding and social connection, which can counteract the effects of cortisol and promote relaxation. Mechanisms and Implications:

The mechanisms underlying the influence of social interactions on cortisol levels are multifaceted. Here are some potential mechanisms and implications:

Stress Buffering:

Social interactions and support networks provide emotional and practical support, which can buffer the impact of stress on cortisol levels. Supportive relationships create a sense of security and promote resilience, helping individuals better cope with stressful situations and reducing the release of cortisol.

Neuroendocrine Pathways:

Social interactions can activate neuroendocrine pathways involved in stress and reward systems. Positive social interactions trigger the release of oxytocin, which has been shown to inhibit the release of cortisol and promote relaxation. In contrast, social isolation and negative interactions can activate stress pathways, leading to cortisol dysregulation.

Psychological Well-being:

Strong social connections contribute to psychological well-being, fostering a sense of belonging, purpose, and self-worth. Positive psychological states have been associated with lower cortisol levels and reduced physiological reactivity to stressors. The emotional support and validation provided by social interactions may help regulate cortisol levels by promoting a sense of safety and reducing the perception of stress.

Health Implications:

Chronic cortisol dysregulation can have implications for physical and mental health. Prolonged exposure to elevated cortisol levels has been associated with adverse health outcomes, including cardiovascular disease, impaired immune function, cognitive decline, and mood disorders. Strong social support networks and positive social interactions may play a protective role by helping to maintain healthy cortisol levels.

So,

The impact of social interactions and support networks on cortisol levels highlights the profound influence of our social lives on our overall well-being. By cultivating positive social connections, fostering supportive relationships, and actively participating in social interactions, we can contribute to the regulation of cortisol levels and promote our own physical and mental health.

Remember, social connections are a two-way street. By offering support, empathy, and compassion to others, we can create a ripple effect of positive social interactions and help mitigate the stress response for both ourselves and those around us. Investing in our social lives can be a powerful tool for stress management, enhancing resilience, and nurturing a sense of belonging and community.

However, it is important to note that each individual's experience may vary, and there are additional factors that can influence cortisol levels. If you are experiencing chronic stress or significant changes in your well-being, it is advisable to consult with healthcare professionals or mental health experts who can provide personalized guidance and support.

Through awareness, understanding, and active participation in meaningful social connections, we can harness the power of social interactions to support healthy cortisol regulation, enhance our overall well-being, and thrive in our interconnected world.

Chapter 63: The Cortisol-Allergic Asthma Connection: Unveiling the Body's Response to Respiratory Allergies

We will explore the intriguing relationship between cortisol and the body's response to allergic asthma. Cortisol, commonly known as the "stress hormone," plays a vital role in our body's stress response and various physiological processes. Allergic asthma, a common respiratory condition, involves airway inflammation triggered by allergens. In this chapter, we will delve into the intricate interplay between cortisol and allergic asthma, shedding light on how cortisol influences the body's response to respiratory allergies and offering insights into potential mechanisms and therapeutic implications.

Understanding Allergic Asthma:

Before we explore the influence of cortisol on allergic asthma, let's establish a foundational understanding of this respiratory condition. Allergic asthma is a chronic inflammatory disorder of the airways characterized by episodes of wheezing, coughing, shortness of breath, and chest tightness. It occurs when the immune system overreacts to harmless substances, such as pollen, dust mites, pet dander, or certain foods, triggering an inflammatory response in the airways.

Cortisol's Impact on the Immune Response in Allergic Asthma:

Cortisol, as a key hormone involved in immune regulation, can modulate the body's response to allergic asthma in various ways. Here's a closer look at its influence:

Anti-inflammatory Effects:

Cortisol has potent anti-inflammatory properties. It suppresses the production and release of pro-inflammatory molecules, such as cytokines and chemokines, thereby reducing airway inflammation in allergic asthma. Corticosteroid medications, which mimic the actions of cortisol, are commonly prescribed to control asthma symptoms, and manage airway inflammation.

Immune Cell Regulation:

Cortisol can modulate the activity of immune cells involved in allergic asthma, such as T cells, mast cells, and eosinophils. It inhibits the activation and recruitment of these cells, leading to a reduction in the release of inflammatory mediators and the subsequent allergic response in the airways.

Airway Smooth Muscle Relaxation:

Cortisol can promote the relaxation of airway smooth muscles, which can help alleviate bronchospasms and improve airflow in allergic asthma. This effect contributes to the management of asthma symptoms and the prevention of asthma attacks.

Epithelial Barrier Function:

The epithelial lining of the airways acts as a barrier against allergens and irritants. Cortisol can enhance the integrity of the epithelial barrier by reducing its permeability and strengthening its protective function. This helps prevent the entry of allergens into the airways and reduces the risk of triggering allergic responses.

Mechanisms and Therapeutic Implications:

The mechanisms underlying cortisol's impact on allergic asthma are multifaceted. Here are some potential mechanisms and therapeutic implications:

Glucocorticoid Receptors:

Cortisol exerts its effects by binding to glucocorticoid receptors present in various cells of the immune system and airways. The activation of these receptors leads to the modulation of gene expression, resulting in anti-inflammatory and immunosuppressive effects. Corticosteroid medications, which mimic cortisol, are often prescribed to enhance glucocorticoid receptor activation and control allergic asthma symptoms.

Timing of Cortisol Release:

The timing of cortisol release in response to allergen exposure is crucial. In healthy individuals, cortisol is naturally released to suppress inflammation and restore homeostasis. However, in some cases, there may be dysregulation in the timing or magnitude of cortisol release, leading to inadequate control of allergic responses. Understanding the dynamics of cortisol release and identifying any abnormalities may help guide therapeutic strategies and optimize asthma management.

Personalized Treatment Approaches:

Individual variations in cortisol levels, sensitivity to corticosteroids, and glucocorticoid receptor expression may contribute to the variability in treatment response among individuals with allergic asthma. Personalized treatment approaches, such as genetic testing or monitoring cortisol levels, may aid in tailoring treatment plans and optimizing therapeutic outcomes.

Lifestyle Factors and Stress Management:

Lifestyle factors, including stress levels, sleep quality, exercise, and nutrition, can impact cortisol levels and the body's response to allergic asthma. Implementing stress management techniques, maintaining a healthy lifestyle, and avoiding triggers can help support cortisol regulation and improve asthma control. However, it is important to note that lifestyle modifications should complement, not replace, medical treatment for allergic asthma.

So,

Cortisol, through its anti-inflammatory effects, immune cell regulation, airway smooth muscle relaxation, and enhancement of epithelial barrier function, plays a significant role in the body's response to allergic asthma. Understanding the intricate interplay between cortisol and allergic asthma can offer valuable insights into the underlying mechanisms and guide therapeutic interventions.

If you or someone you know has allergic asthma, it is important to work closely with healthcare professionals to develop a comprehensive management plan. This plan may include medications, such as corticosteroids, bronchodilators, and immunomodulators, as well as lifestyle modifications and trigger avoidance strategies.

By harnessing the anti-inflammatory and immunosuppressive properties of cortisol, healthcare providers can optimize treatment strategies and help individuals with allergic asthma achieve better control of their symptoms, improve lung function, and enhance their overall quality of life.

Remember, the information provided in this chapter is intended to offer a deeper understanding of the relationship between cortisol and allergic asthma. It should not replace professional medical advice or treatment. If you have any questions or concerns about your specific condition, consult with your healthcare provider, who can provide personalized guidance based on your unique needs and circumstances. With continued research and a comprehensive approach to allergic asthma management, we can strive to reduce the burden of this respiratory condition and empower individuals to live healthier, more fulfilling lives.

Chapter 64: Unveiling the Cortisol-Pollutant Connection: Exploring the Impact of Environmental Pollutants on the Body's Stress Response

We will delve into the intriguing relationship between cortisol and the body's response to environmental pollutants. Cortisol, commonly known as the "stress hormone," plays a vital role in our body's stress response and various physiological processes. Environmental pollutants, such as air pollution, chemicals, heavy metals, and pesticides, pose significant risks to our health and well-being. In this chapter, we will explore the intricate interplay between cortisol and environmental pollutants, shedding light on how cortisol impacts the body's response to these pollutants and offering insights into the potential implications for our health and strategies for mitigating their effects.

Understanding Environmental Pollutants:

Before we explore the influence of cortisol on environmental pollutants, let's establish a foundational understanding of these pollutants. Environmental pollutants refer to substances released into the environment that can cause harm to living organisms. They can originate from various sources, including industrial emissions, vehicle exhaust, agricultural activities, and household chemicals. Common types of environmental pollutants include particulate matter, volatile organic compounds (VOCs), heavy metals, ozone, and persistent organic pollutants (POPs).

Cortisol's Role in the Body's Stress Response:

Cortisol is a hormone produced by the adrenal glands in response to stress. It plays a vital role in our body's stress response and helps regulate various physiological processes. When we encounter stressful situations, cortisol is released into our bloodstream, preparing our bodies for a "fight or flight" response. However, prolonged, or chronic exposure to stress can lead to dysregulation of cortisol levels, potentially impacting our health.

Cortisol and the Impact of Environmental Pollutants:

Environmental pollutants can elicit stress responses in the body, triggering the release of cortisol. Here's a closer look at how cortisol interacts with different types of pollutants:

Air Pollution:

Air pollution, including particulate matter and VOCs, has been linked to increased cortisol levels. Inhalation of polluted air can activate inflammatory responses in the respiratory system, leading to oxidative stress and tissue damage. This activation of the immune system can trigger the release of cortisol as part of the body's stress response.

Heavy Metals:

Exposure to heavy metals, such as lead, mercury, arsenic, and cadmium, can disrupt the body's stress response and cortisol regulation. Heavy metals have toxic effects on various organs and can impair the function of the hypothalamic-pituitary-adrenal (HPA) axis, which controls cortisol release. Dysregulation of cortisol levels due to heavy metal exposure can further contribute to oxidative stress, inflammation, and organ damage.

Pesticides and Chemicals:

Certain pesticides and chemicals, such as organophosphates and bisphenol A (BPA), have been associated with altered cortisol levels. These substances can interfere with hormone signaling pathways, including the HPA axis, leading to cortisol dysregulation. Prolonged exposure to pesticides and chemicals can disrupt the body's ability to respond to stress appropriately, impacting overall health and well-being.

Mechanisms and Strategies for Mitigating the Effects:

The mechanisms underlying cortisol's impact on the body's response to environmental pollutants are complex. Here are some potential mechanisms and strategies for mitigating their effects:

Oxidative Stress and Inflammation:

Environmental pollutants can induce oxidative stress and inflammation in the body. Cortisol plays a role in modulating these processes by exerting anti-inflammatory effects and regulating the expression of antioxidant enzymes. Maintaining balanced cortisol levels and supporting antioxidant defense mechanisms through a healthy lifestyle, including a nutritious diet rich in antioxidants, regular exercise, and stress management, can help mitigate the oxidative stress and inflammation induced by pollutants.

Detoxification Pathways:

Environmental pollutants can accumulate in the body over time, leading to toxic burden. Cortisol is involved in detoxification processes by activating enzymes responsible for the metabolism and elimination of toxins. Enhancing the body's natural detoxification pathways through proper nutrition, hydration, and lifestyle choices can support cortisol's role in detoxification and help reduce the adverse effects of environmental pollutants.

Supportive Measures:

Reducing exposure to environmental pollutants is crucial for minimizing their impact on cortisol levels and overall health. Taking preventive measures, such as using air purifiers, practicing proper ventilation, using natural and eco-friendly cleaning products, and consuming organic foods, can help limit exposure to pollutants. Additionally, engaging in stress reduction techniques, such as mindfulness, meditation, and relaxation exercises, can support cortisol regulation and enhance the body's resilience to environmental stressors.

So,

The interplay between cortisol and environmental pollutants highlights the importance of understanding the impact of our surroundings on our health. Environmental pollutants can disrupt cortisol regulation, leading to systemic inflammation, oxidative stress, and various health concerns. By adopting a proactive approach that combines environmental awareness, pollutant reduction strategies, and stress management techniques, we can mitigate the effects of environmental pollutants on cortisol levels and promote our overall well-being.

It is essential to stay informed about local environmental conditions, seek guidance from relevant authorities, and make conscious choices to protect ourselves and the environment. Additionally, consulting with healthcare professionals can provide personalized advice and guidance based on individual circumstances.

Through collective efforts, public awareness, and responsible environmental stewardship, we can create a healthier and more sustainable environment for future generations, where the impact of environmental pollutants on cortisol levels and overall health is minimized.

Chapter 65: The Cortisol-Kidney Connection: Exploring the Impact of Cortisol on Kidney Health

We will delve into the fascinating relationship between cortisol and kidney diseases. Cortisol, commonly known as the "stress hormone," plays a vital role in our body's stress response and various physiological processes. The kidneys, on the other hand, play a crucial role in maintaining our overall health by filtering waste products, regulating fluid balance, and producing hormones. In this chapter, we will explore the intricate interplay between cortisol and kidney health, shedding light on how cortisol impacts the development and progression of kidney diseases and offering insights into potential mechanisms and therapeutic implications.

Understanding Kidney Diseases:

Before we explore the influence of cortisol on kidney diseases, let's establish a foundational understanding of these conditions. Kidney diseases encompass a broad range of disorders that affect the structure and function of the kidneys. Common types of kidney diseases include chronic kidney disease (CKD), acute kidney injury (AKI), polycystic kidney disease (PKD), and glomerulonephritis. These conditions can impair the kidneys' ability to filter waste products, maintain electrolyte balance, regulate blood pressure, and produce essential hormones.

Cortisol's Impact on Kidney Health:

Cortisol can influence kidney health through various mechanisms. Here's a closer look at its impact on kidney function and the development and progression of kidney diseases:

Glucocorticoid Receptor Activation:

Cortisol binds to glucocorticoid receptors present in the kidneys, affecting their function and the regulation of fluid and electrolyte balance. Activation of these receptors can lead to sodium and water retention, increased blood pressure, and altered electrolyte levels. Prolonged activation of glucocorticoid receptors due to elevated cortisol levels or excessive exogenous glucocorticoid administration can contribute to the development of kidney diseases.

Inflammation and Fibrosis:

Cortisol plays a role in modulating inflammation and fibrosis, which are key processes involved in the progression of kidney diseases. Elevated cortisol levels can promote inflammation in the kidneys, leading to immune cell infiltration, oxidative stress, and tissue damage. Chronic inflammation can contribute to the development of fibrosis, a process characterized by the excessive deposition of extracellular matrix components in the kidneys. Fibrosis can impair kidney function and contribute to the progression of kidney diseases.

Blood Pressure Regulation:

Cortisol, through its impact on blood pressure regulation, can indirectly influence kidney health. Elevated cortisol levels can lead to increased blood pressure by promoting sodium and water retention, vasoconstriction, and the activation of the renin-angiotensin-aldosterone system. High blood pressure, or hypertension, is a significant risk factor for the development and progression of kidney diseases, including CKD and glomerulonephritis.

Glucose Metabolism and Diabetes:

Cortisol is involved in glucose metabolism, and elevated cortisol levels can contribute to insulin resistance and impaired glucose control. Diabetes, a condition characterized by elevated blood glucose levels, is a major risk factor for the development of CKD. The interplay between cortisol, glucose metabolism, and diabetes can impact kidney health, as chronic hyperglycemia can damage the blood vessels and structures in the kidneys.

Mechanisms and Therapeutic Implications:

The mechanisms underlying cortisol's impact on kidney health are complex. Here are some potential mechanisms and therapeutic implications:

Glucocorticoid Receptor Modulation:

Targeting glucocorticoid receptors in the kidneys may be a potential therapeutic approach for managing kidney diseases. Selective glucocorticoid receptor modulators, which can specifically activate or inhibit these receptors in a tissue-specific manner, could help mitigate the adverse effects of cortisol on kidney function and inflammation.

Inflammation and Fibrosis Control:

Strategies that target inflammation and fibrosis may offer therapeutic benefits for kidney diseases influenced by cortisol. Anti-inflammatory agents, such as corticosteroids or immunomodulatory drugs, can help mitigate inflammation in the kidneys. Inhibitors targeting fibrotic pathways, such as transforming growth factor-beta (TGF-β) inhibitors or specific matrix metalloproteinase (MMP) inhibitors, may help prevent or slow down fibrosis progression.

Blood Pressure Management:

Controlling blood pressure is crucial for maintaining kidney health. Lifestyle modifications, including a balanced diet low in sodium, regular physical activity, and stress management techniques, can help regulate blood pressure and minimize the impact of cortisol-induced hypertension on kidney function. Medications that target the renin-angiotensin-aldosterone system, such as angiotensin-converting enzyme (ACE) inhibitors or angiotensin receptor blockers (ARBs), may also be prescribed to manage hypertension and protect kidney function.

Diabetes Management:

Managing diabetes effectively is essential for preventing or managing kidney diseases influenced by cortisol. Tight glycemic control through diet, exercise, medication, and regular monitoring can help reduce the risk of kidney complications associated with diabetes. Additionally, medications targeting specific pathways involved in glucose metabolism, such as sodium-glucose cotransporter-2 (SGLT-2) inhibitors, may have additional benefits for kidney health.
So,
The intricate relationship between cortisol and kidney diseases highlights the importance of understanding the impact of cortisol on kidney health and exploring therapeutic interventions to mitigate its adverse effects. Cortisol, through its influence on glucocorticoid receptors, inflammation, fibrosis, blood pressure regulation, and glucose metabolism, can contribute to the development and progression of kidney diseases. By targeting these mechanisms through

personalized treatment approaches, such as glucocorticoid receptor modulation, inflammation and fibrosis control, blood pressure management, and diabetes management, healthcare professionals can optimize therapeutic strategies and improve kidney health outcomes.

It is crucial for individuals with kidney diseases or those at risk to work closely with healthcare professionals who can provide personalized guidance and monitoring. Regular kidney function assessments, adherence to treatment plans, lifestyle modifications, and close management of underlying conditions, such as hypertension or diabetes, are essential for maintaining kidney health.

Through continued research, advancements in personalized medicine, and comprehensive management approaches, we can strive to better understand the intricate interplay between cortisol and kidney diseases. By unraveling the mechanisms involved and developing targeted therapeutic strategies, we can improve outcomes for individuals with kidney diseases and enhance their quality of life.

It's important to note that the information provided in this chapter is intended to offer a deeper understanding of the relationship between cortisol and kidney diseases. It should not replace professional medical advice or treatment. If you have any concerns about your kidney health or specific conditions, consult with your healthcare provider, who can provide personalized guidance based on your unique needs and circumstances.

With a holistic approach that combines medical interventions, lifestyle modifications, and regular monitoring, we can work towards better managing kidney diseases and minimizing the impact of cortisol on kidney health. By fostering awareness, promoting kidney health education, and supporting ongoing research, we can make significant strides in preventing, managing, and treating kidney diseases for a healthier future.

Chapter 66: The Cortisol-Air Pollution Connection: Exploring the Impact of Air Pollution and Smog on Cortisol Levels

We will dive into the intriguing relationship between cortisol and exposure to air pollution and smog. Air pollution, a global environmental challenge, poses significant risks to our health and well-being. Cortisol, commonly known as the "stress hormone," plays a vital role in our body's stress response and various physiological processes. In this chapter, we will explore the intricate interplay between cortisol and air pollution, shedding light on how exposure to air pollution and smog can influence cortisol levels and the potential implications for our health.

Understanding Air Pollution and Smog:

Before we delve into the influence of air pollution on cortisol levels, let's establish a foundational understanding of air pollution and smog. Air pollution refers to the presence of harmful substances in the air, resulting from various sources such as vehicle emissions, industrial processes, and the burning of fossil fuels. These pollutants can include particulate matter, nitrogen dioxide, sulfur dioxide, ozone, and volatile organic compounds. When air pollution reaches high levels, it can create a visible haze known as smog, which is a combination of pollutants that can negatively impact air quality and human health.

The Impact of Air Pollution on Cortisol Levels:

Exposure to air pollution and smog can trigger physiological responses in the body, including the release of cortisol. Here's a closer look at how air pollution can influence cortisol levels:

Inflammation and Oxidative Stress:

Air pollution is known to induce inflammation and oxidative stress in the body. When we breathe in polluted air, harmful particles, such as fine particulate matter (PM2.5) and toxic gases, can penetrate deep into our respiratory system. This triggers an immune response, leading to the release of pro-inflammatory cytokines and the generation of reactive oxygen species. In response to this inflammation and oxidative stress, cortisol levels may rise as part of the body's stress response.

Autonomic Nervous System Activation:

Exposure to air pollution can activate the autonomic nervous system, which regulates involuntary bodily functions. This activation is often observed as an increase in sympathetic nervous system activity, commonly known as the "fight or flight" response. This response can lead to an elevation in cortisol levels, as cortisol is one of the hormones involved in the body's stress response.

Psychological Stress:

Living in areas with high levels of air pollution can also induce psychological stress. The visible haze, foul odor, and knowledge of the potential health risks associated with air pollution can contribute to increased anxiety and stress levels. Psychological stress, whether directly related to air pollution or the concern for its impact, can influence cortisol secretion and contribute to elevated cortisol levels.

Health Implications and Considerations:

The impact of elevated cortisol levels due to exposure to air pollution and smog can have several health implications. Here are some considerations:

Respiratory Health:

Air pollution, particularly fine particulate matter, can irritate the respiratory system, trigger asthma attacks, worsen chronic obstructive pulmonary disease (COPD), and increase the risk of respiratory infections. Prolonged exposure to polluted air and the subsequent elevation in cortisol levels may further exacerbate these conditions and impact overall respiratory health.

Cardiovascular Health:

Air pollution is a well-known risk factor for cardiovascular diseases such as heart attacks, strokes, and hypertension. Elevated cortisol levels due to exposure to air pollution can contribute to increased blood pressure, inflammation, and oxidative stress, which are all factors implicated in the development and progression of cardiovascular diseases.

Immune Function:

Cortisol, as a key regulator of the immune system, plays a vital role in modulating immune responses. Elevated cortisol levels induced by air pollution can have immunosuppressive effects, compromising the body's ability to fight infections and increasing susceptibility to respiratory illnesses.

Mental Well-being:

Exposure to air pollution and the subsequent elevation in cortisol levels can also impact mental well-being. Research suggests a potential link between air pollution and psychological distress, including symptoms of anxiety and depression. Chronic exposure to polluted air may contribute to long-term psychological stress, further impacting mental health and overall well-being.

Mitigating the Effects of Air Pollution:

While we may not have direct control over air pollution levels, there are steps we can take to mitigate the effects and reduce exposure. Consider the following strategies:

Monitor Air Quality:

Stay informed about air quality conditions in your area by accessing local air quality indexes and alerts. Limit outdoor activities during periods of high pollution and take necessary precautions to protect yourself and your family.

Create Indoor Sanctuaries:

Improve indoor air quality by ensuring proper ventilation, using air purifiers or filters, and minimizing the use of household products that release pollutants. Creating a clean and healthy indoor environment can provide a sanctuary from outdoor pollution.

Practice Protective Measures:

When air pollution levels are high, take extra precautions to protect your respiratory system. Wear masks designed to filter out fine particles (N95 masks) during outdoor activities, especially in heavily polluted areas or when engaged in physical exertion.

Support Clean Air Initiatives:

Advocate for clean air policies and support initiatives aimed at reducing air pollution. Encourage the use of cleaner energy sources, promote sustainable transportation options, and participate in community efforts to improve air quality.

So,

The relationship between cortisol and exposure to air pollution and smog highlights the complex interplay between our environment and our health. Air pollution can trigger physiological responses in the body, including an increase in cortisol levels. Elevated cortisol levels due to air pollution exposure can have various implications for respiratory health, cardiovascular health, immune function, and mental well-being.

While we continue to work towards improving air quality on a global scale, it is essential to prioritize personal measures to reduce exposure and mitigate the effects of air pollution. By staying informed, creating clean indoor environments, practicing protective measures, and supporting clean air initiatives, we can minimize the impact of air pollution on cortisol levels and protect our health and well-being.

Remember, this chapter is intended to provide insights into the relationship between cortisol and air pollution, but it should not replace professional medical advice or environmental guidance. If you have specific concerns about your health or air quality conditions in your area, consult with healthcare professionals and relevant environmental agencies who can provide tailored advice based on your circumstances.

Together, through collective efforts and a commitment to environmental stewardship, we can create cleaner and healthier environments for ourselves and future generations.

Chapter 67: Cortisol and Radiation Exposure: Understanding the Body's Response

We will explore the fascinating relationship between cortisol and the body's response to radiation exposure. Radiation is a form of energy that can have both beneficial and harmful effects on living organisms. Cortisol, commonly known as the "stress hormone," plays a crucial role in our body's stress response and various physiological processes. In this chapter, we will delve into the impact of cortisol on the body's response to radiation exposure, shedding light on how cortisol levels can be influenced and the potential implications for our health.

Understanding Radiation Exposure:

Before we explore the influence of cortisol on radiation exposure, let's establish a foundational understanding of radiation and its effects on the human body. Radiation can be categorized into two types: ionizing radiation and non-ionizing radiation. Ionizing radiation, such as X-rays, gamma rays, and certain types of particles, has sufficient energy to remove tightly bound electrons from atoms, leading to potential damage to biological tissues. Non-ionizing radiation, such as radio waves and visible light, has lower energy levels and is generally considered less harmful.

The Impact of Cortisol on Radiation Exposure:

Radiation exposure can induce physiological responses in the body, including the release of cortisol. Here's a closer look at how cortisol can influence the body's response to radiation exposure:

Stress Response Activation:

Radiation exposure is a stressful event for the body, triggering the activation of the stress response system. In response to stress, the adrenal glands release cortisol, which helps the body cope with the physiological and psychological demands of the situation. Cortisol mobilizes energy reserves, enhances alertness, and modulates immune and inflammatory responses. Therefore, radiation exposure can lead to an increase in cortisol levels as part of the body's natural stress response.

Inflammation and Tissue Damage:

Radiation exposure can cause tissue damage through various mechanisms, including the production of reactive oxygen species (ROS) and the activation of inflammatory pathways. Cortisol, as an anti-inflammatory hormone, helps regulate the body's inflammatory response. Elevated cortisol levels during radiation exposure can modulate inflammation and potentially mitigate some of the inflammatory processes associated with tissue damage.

Immune System Modulation:

The immune system plays a critical role in responding to radiation-induced tissue damage. Cortisol, as an immunomodulatory hormone, can influence the immune response to radiation exposure. High cortisol levels may have immunosuppressive effects, potentially impacting the immune system's ability to repair damaged tissues and fight off infections that may arise from radiation exposure.

DNA Repair and Cell Survival:

Radiation exposure can cause DNA damage within cells. The body has sophisticated mechanisms to repair this damage and promote cell survival. Cortisol can influence these processes by modulating gene expression and cellular signaling pathways involved in DNA repair. Elevated cortisol levels may support the body's DNA repair mechanisms, enhancing cell survival and potentially minimizing the long-term effects of radiation exposure.

Radiation Therapy and Cortisol:

It's important to note that the impact of cortisol on radiation exposure can vary depending on the context. In radiation therapy, for example, cortisol can have both beneficial and challenging effects:

Sensitizing Effect:

In some cases, cortisol administration before radiation therapy may enhance the sensitivity of tumor cells to radiation. This sensitizing effect aims to improve the therapeutic response and increase the effectiveness of radiation treatment. However, the precise mechanisms and optimal strategies for cortisol administration in conjunction with radiation therapy require further research and careful consideration.

Side Effects:

While cortisol can enhance the sensitivity of tumor cells to radiation, it may also have some adverse effects on healthy tissues. Cortisol's immunosuppressive properties can impact the normal tissue response to radiation, potentially leading to increased vulnerability to radiation-induced side effects. Therefore, finding the right balance between enhancing therapeutic efficacy and minimizing side effects remains a challenge in radiation therapy.

So,

The relationship between cortisol and the body's response to radiation exposure highlights the complexity of radiation's effects on human physiology. Cortisol, as a key hormone in the stress response, can influence the body's reaction to radiation exposure through stress response activation, inflammation modulation, immune system modulation, and DNA repair facilitation. However, the precise role of cortisol in radiation response requires further investigation, and its impact may depend on various factors such as radiation dose, duration of exposure, and individual differences.

It's important to note that this chapter provides insights into the influence of cortisol on radiation exposure, but it should not replace professional medical advice or radiation therapy guidelines. If you have specific concerns about radiation exposure or treatment, consult with healthcare professionals who can provide personalized guidance based on your unique circumstances.

As researchers continue to investigate the intricate interplay between cortisol and radiation exposure, further advancements in personalized medicine and radiation therapy techniques may emerge. By optimizing treatment strategies, considering the potential impact of cortisol, and minimizing radiation-induced side effects, we can work towards improving the outcomes for individuals undergoing radiation therapy or facing radiation exposure.

Together, through ongoing research, multidisciplinary collaboration, and a commitment to patient-centered care, we can deepen our understanding of the complex relationship between cortisol and radiation exposure, paving the way for more effective and personalized approaches to radiation therapy and radiation protection.

Chapter 68: Navigating Menopause: Exploring the Influence of Cortisol on Hormonal Changes

We will delve into the fascinating relationship between cortisol and the body's response to hormonal changes during menopause. Menopause is a natural biological process that marks the end of a woman's reproductive years. It brings about significant hormonal shifts, including a decline in estrogen and progesterone levels. Cortisol, known as the "stress hormone," plays a crucial role in our body's stress response and various physiological processes. In this chapter, we will explore how cortisol can impact the body's response to hormonal changes during menopause and discuss potential implications for women's health.

Understanding Menopause and Hormonal Changes:

Before we explore the influence of cortisol on menopause, let's establish a foundational understanding of menopause and the hormonal changes that occur. Menopause typically occurs in women between the ages of 45 and 55, although the timing can vary. During menopause, the ovaries gradually produce fewer reproductive hormones, leading to the cessation of menstrual periods and the end of fertility. The decline in estrogen and progesterone levels during menopause can give rise to various physical and emotional symptoms.

The Impact of Cortisol on Menopause:

Cortisol can influence the body's response to hormonal changes during menopause in several ways:

Stress Response and Symptom Perception:

Menopause is a transitional phase that can be accompanied by increased stress levels due to various factors such as physical discomfort, emotional changes, and lifestyle adjustments. Cortisol, as a key hormone involved in the stress response, can impact how women perceive and experience menopausal symptoms. Higher cortisol levels during periods of stress may contribute to increased symptom intensity, such as hot flashes, mood swings, and sleep disturbances.

Hormonal Balance and Estrogen Metabolism:

Cortisol and estrogen share complex interactions within the body. Elevated cortisol levels can influence estrogen metabolism, potentially leading to imbalances in estrogen levels. Cortisol can affect enzymes involved in estrogen metabolism, which may result in alterations in estrogen synthesis, clearance, and the ratio of active estrogen metabolites. These changes in estrogen metabolism may contribute to the onset or exacerbation of menopausal symptoms.

Bone Health and Osteoporosis Risk:

Estrogen plays a crucial role in maintaining bone health, and the decline in estrogen levels during menopause can increase the risk of osteoporosis. Cortisol, when present in excess or dysregulated levels, can have detrimental effects on bone health. High cortisol levels may interfere with bone remodeling, leading to decreased bone density and an increased risk of fractures. The interplay between cortisol and estrogen in the context of bone health during menopause is a complex area that requires further research.

Emotional Well-being and Mental Health:

Menopause is often accompanied by emotional changes, including mood swings, anxiety, and depression. Cortisol, as a hormone involved in stress regulation, can impact emotional well-being and mental health. Dysregulation of cortisol levels, such as chronically elevated or suppressed cortisol, may contribute to mood disturbances and psychological symptoms during menopause. It's important to note that individual variations and other factors, such as personal history, lifestyle, and social support, can also influence emotional well-being during this transitional phase.

Coping Strategies and Support:

While we cannot control the natural hormonal changes of menopause or eliminate the impact of cortisol, there are strategies and support systems that can help women navigate this phase with greater ease:

Stress Management Techniques:

Implement stress management techniques, such as relaxation exercises, mindfulness, deep breathing, and engaging in activities that promote relaxation and emotional well-being. These techniques can help regulate cortisol levels and alleviate stress-related symptoms during menopause.

Regular Exercise:

Engage in regular physical activity, as it can have multiple benefits during menopause. Exercise can help reduce stress, improve mood, support bone health, and contribute to overall well-being. Consult with healthcare professionals to determine the most suitable exercise regimen for your needs and capabilities.

Healthy Lifestyle Choices:

Adopt a healthy lifestyle that includes a balanced diet rich in nutrients, regular sleep patterns, and avoidance of excessive ... consumption and tobacco use. These lifestyle choices can positively impact hormonal balance, overall health, and well-being during menopause.

Seek Support and Education:

Connect with support networks, such as menopause support groups, where you can share experiences, seek advice, and gain knowledge about menopause. Education and understanding can empower you to make informed decisions about your health and seek appropriate medical care when needed.

So,

Menopause is a significant life transition for women, marked by hormonal changes that can impact physical and emotional well-being. The influence of cortisol on menopause adds another layer of complexity to this transformative phase. Cortisol, as a stress-regulating hormone, can influence how menopausal symptoms are experienced, impact hormonal balance, bone health, and emotional well-being.

While we cannot control the natural hormonal changes or eliminate the impact of cortisol, we can take steps to support our overall well-being during menopause. By practicing stress management techniques, engaging in regular exercise, making healthy lifestyle choices, and seeking support and education, women can navigate this phase with greater resilience and enhanced quality of life.

It's important to note that this chapter provides insights into the relationship between cortisol and menopause, but it should not replace professional medical advice or treatment. If you have specific concerns or questions about menopause or related symptoms, consult with healthcare professionals who can provide personalized guidance based on your unique circumstances.

Through a holistic approach that combines self-care, informed decision-making, and access to appropriate medical care, women can embrace menopause as a transformative journey and cultivate well-being and vitality during this new chapter of life.

Chapter 69: Unveiling the Connection Between Cortisol and Liver Diseases

We will embark on an exploration of the relationship between cortisol and liver diseases. The liver is an essential organ involved in numerous metabolic processes, including detoxification, nutrient metabolism, and hormone regulation. Cortisol, often referred to as the "stress hormone," plays a vital role in the body's stress response and has diverse effects on various organ systems. In this chapter, we will delve into the influence of cortisol on the development and progression of liver diseases, shedding light on the complex interplay between this hormone and liver health.

Understanding Liver Diseases:

Before we delve into the role of cortisol, let's establish a foundational understanding of liver diseases. Liver diseases encompass a broad spectrum of conditions that affect the structure and function of the liver. These diseases can range from viral infections, such as hepatitis, to chronic conditions like cirrhosis and liver cancer. Liver diseases can be influenced by various factors, including genetics, lifestyle choices, exposure to toxins, and certain medical conditions.

The Impact of Cortisol on Liver Diseases:

Cortisol can exert both beneficial and detrimental effects on the liver, depending on the context and duration of exposure. Here's a closer look at the influence of cortisol on the development and progression of liver diseases:

Metabolism and Fat Accumulation:

Cortisol can affect liver metabolism and contribute to the accumulation of fat in the liver, a condition known as (NAFLD). Elevated cortisol levels can stimulate the breakdown of muscle proteins, leading to increased amino acid availability. These amino acids can be converted into glucose through a process called gluconeogenesis. Prolonged elevation of cortisol levels and increased gluconeogenesis can result in elevated blood glucose levels and an increased risk of developing NAFLD.

Inflammation and Fibrosis:

Chronic liver diseases, such as viral hepatitis often involve persistent inflammation and the development of fibrosis, which can progress to cirrhosis. Cortisol, as an anti-inflammatory hormone, has the potential to modulate the liver's inflammatory response. However, sustained high levels of cortisol can impair the resolution of inflammation and promote the development of fibrosis, exacerbating liver damage.

Immune Function and Autoimmune Hepatitis:

Autoimmune hepatitis is a liver disease characterized by an abnormal immune response that targets the liver cells. Cortisol has immunosuppressive effects and can regulate the immune response. In autoimmune hepatitis, dysregulation of cortisol levels or altered cortisol sensitivity may contribute to the loss of immune tolerance and the development of autoimmunity. Further research is needed to fully understand the role of cortisol in autoimmune hepatitis.

Drug Metabolism and Hepatotoxicity:

The liver plays a critical role in drug metabolism and detoxification. Cortisol can influence liver enzyme activity involved in drug metabolism, potentially affecting the clearance and efficacy of certain medications. Moreover, in some cases, prolonged exposure to high cortisol levels can increase the susceptibility of liver cells to drug-induced damage, leading to hepatotoxicity.

Managing Cortisol Levels and Liver Health:

While we cannot completely control cortisol levels or prevent all liver diseases, there are strategies that can support liver health and potentially mitigate the impact of cortisol:

Stress Management:

Effective stress management techniques, such as relaxation exercises, mindfulness, and engaging in enjoyable activities, can help regulate cortisol levels and reduce the impact of chronic stress on the liver. Implementing stress reduction techniques can promote overall well-being and support liver health.

Healthy Lifestyle Choices:

Adopting a healthy lifestyle is crucial for liver health. This includes maintaining a balanced diet rich in fruits, vegetables, and whole grains, while minimizing the consumption of processed foods,

..., and other substances that can negatively impact liver function. Regular exercise, adequate sleep, and avoiding exposure to toxins can also contribute to liver health.

Medication and Treatment Monitoring:

If you are taking medications that may affect liver function, it is important to discuss with your healthcare provider regularly and undergo routine liver function tests. Monitoring liver enzyme levels can help identify any potential medication-related liver issues.

Regular Medical Check-ups:

Regular check-ups with your healthcare provider allow for the early detection and management of liver diseases. This is particularly important if you have underlying conditions that may increase your risk of liver disease or if you have a family history of liver disorders.

So,

Understanding the complex relationship between cortisol and liver diseases is an ongoing area of research. While cortisol plays a significant role in the body's stress response and can impact liver health, the precise mechanisms, and the extent of its influence on specific liver diseases require further investigation.

Taking proactive steps to support liver health, such as practicing stress management techniques, adopting a healthy lifestyle, and monitoring medication use, can contribute to overall well-being and potentially mitigate the impact of cortisol on liver health. However, it is crucial to seek guidance from healthcare professionals for personalized advice and treatment options tailored to your unique circumstances.

By combining knowledge, research advancements, and a commitment to liver health, we can work towards a comprehensive understanding of the interplay between cortisol and liver diseases. Through ongoing research, preventive measures, and early interventions, we can strive to improve liver health outcomes and enhance the well-being of individuals affected by liver diseases.

Chapter 70: Unveiling the Impact of Heavy Metals and Toxins on Cortisol Levels

We will explore the intriguing relationship between exposure to heavy metals and toxins and cortisol levels. Heavy metals and toxins are ubiquitous in our environment and can have detrimental effects on human health. Cortisol, often referred to as the "stress hormone," plays a vital role in our body's stress response and various physiological processes. In this chapter, we will delve into how exposure to heavy metals and toxins can influence cortisol levels, shedding light on the complex interplay between these toxic substances and our hormonal balance.

Understanding Heavy Metals and Toxins:

Before we dive into the impact on cortisol levels, let's establish a foundational understanding of heavy metals and toxins. Heavy metals, such as lead, mercury, cadmium, and arsenic, are naturally occurring elements with high atomic weights. They can enter the environment through various industrial processes, pollution, and certain products. Toxins, on the other hand, encompass a wide range of harmful substances, including pesticides, industrial chemicals, pollutants, and certain medications. Both heavy metals and toxins have the potential to accumulate in our bodies and cause adverse health effects.

The Influence of Heavy Metals and Toxins on Cortisol Levels:

Exposure to heavy metals and toxins can affect cortisol levels in several ways:

Activation of the Stress Response:

Exposure to heavy metals and toxins can trigger a stress response in the body, leading to an increase in cortisol levels. The presence of these toxic substances activates the body's defense mechanisms, resulting in the release of stress hormones, including cortisol. This stress response aims to mobilize energy, enhance alertness, and initiate detoxification processes to counteract the harmful effects of heavy metals and toxins.

Disruption of Hormonal Regulation:

Heavy metals and toxins can disrupt the delicate balance of hormonal regulation in the body, including the regulation of cortisol. These substances can interfere with the function of the endocrine system, which controls hormone production and secretion. The disruption of hormonal regulation can lead to dysregulation of cortisol levels, resulting in either elevated or suppressed cortisol production.

Oxidative Stress and Inflammation:

Exposure to heavy metals and toxins can induce oxidative stress and inflammation in the body. Oxidative stress occurs when there is an imbalance between the production of harmful free radicals and the body's antioxidant defenses. This imbalance can activate inflammatory pathways, leading to the release of pro-inflammatory cytokines. Both oxidative stress and inflammation can impact cortisol levels, potentially leading to an imbalance in cortisol production.

Impact on the HPA Axis:

The hypothalamic-pituitary-adrenal (HPA) axis is a crucial system involved in the regulation of cortisol. Heavy metals and toxins can disrupt the HPA axis, leading to alterations in cortisol levels. These substances can affect the function of the hypothalamus and pituitary gland, which control cortisol release from the adrenal glands. Disruption of the HPA axis can result in abnormal cortisol production and dysregulated stress response.

Managing Heavy Metal and Toxin Exposure:

While it may be challenging to completely avoid exposure to heavy metals and toxins, there are measures we can take to minimize their impact and support our overall well-being:

Reduce Exposure:

Be mindful of potential sources of heavy metals and toxins in your environment. This includes avoiding contaminated foods, using safe and non-toxic household products, filtering drinking water, and minimizing exposure to pollutants and industrial chemicals. Adhering to proper safety measures and following recommended guidelines can help reduce exposure to these harmful substances.

Detoxification Support:

Support your body's natural detoxification processes by adopting a healthy lifestyle. This includes consuming a nutrient-rich diet, staying adequately hydrated, engaging in regular physical activity, and getting sufficient sleep. These practices can enhance your body's ability to eliminate toxins and support overall well-being.

Antioxidant-Rich Diet:

Include antioxidant-rich foods in your diet, such as fruits, vegetables, nuts, and seeds. Antioxidants help neutralize free radicals and reduce oxidative stress. By supporting your body's antioxidant defenses, you can mitigate the potential harmful effects of heavy metals and toxins.

Seek Professional Guidance:

If you suspect heavy metal or toxin exposure or experience symptoms associated with toxicity, consult with healthcare professionals who specialize in environmental medicine or toxicology. They can provide guidance, conduct appropriate testing, and recommend individualized detoxification protocols if necessary.

So,

Exposure to heavy metals and toxins can influence cortisol levels and disrupt the delicate balance of our hormonal regulation. While it may be challenging to completely avoid exposure, adopting preventive measures and supporting our body's natural detoxification processes can help mitigate the potential impact of these harmful substances.

It's essential to stay informed, be mindful of potential sources of heavy metals and toxins and seek professional guidance if needed. By taking proactive steps to reduce exposure, support our body's natural detoxification mechanisms, and prioritize overall well-being, we can strive to minimize the potential disruption to cortisol levels and promote a healthier, more balanced hormonal environment.

Please note that this chapter provides insights into the relationship between heavy metals, toxins, and cortisol levels. However, it should not replace professional medical advice or assessment. If you have specific concerns or suspect heavy metal or toxin exposure, consult with healthcare professionals who can provide personalized guidance based on your unique circumstances.

Chapter 71: Unraveling the Connection Between Cortisol and Autoimmune Hepatitis

We will embark on an exploration of the relationship between cortisol and the body's response to autoimmune hepatitis. Autoimmune hepatitis is a chronic liver disease characterized by inflammation and damage to liver cells caused by an abnormal immune response. Cortisol, often referred to as the "stress hormone," plays a crucial role in immune regulation and the body's response to stress. In this chapter, we will delve into the influence of cortisol on the development and progression of autoimmune hepatitis, shedding light on the intricate interplay between this hormone and the immune system in the context of liver health.

Understanding Autoimmune Hepatitis:

Before we delve into the role of cortisol, let's establish a foundational understanding of autoimmune hepatitis. This condition occurs when the immune system mistakenly identifies liver cells as foreign and launches an immune attack against them. Over time, this immune response leads to inflammation, damage, and, if left untreated, can progress to fibrosis and cirrhosis. Autoimmune hepatitis is considered a complex disorder influenced by genetic predisposition and environmental factors, though its exact cause remains unknown.

The Impact of Cortisol on Autoimmune Hepatitis:

Cortisol, as a key player in immune regulation, can influence the development and progression of autoimmune hepatitis in several ways:

Immune Modulation:

Cortisol possesses potent immunosuppressive properties that help regulate the immune system and prevent excessive inflammation. In the context of autoimmune hepatitis, elevated cortisol levels may serve as an attempt to suppress the immune response, thereby reducing the ongoing liver inflammation. However, it is important to note that the immune dysregulation observed in autoimmune hepatitis may involve complex interactions between cortisol and other immune-regulating molecules.

Cortisol Sensitivity:

In some individuals with autoimmune hepatitis, alterations in cortisol sensitivity or cortisol receptor function may contribute to the development or progression of the disease. Abnormalities in cortisol receptor signaling can affect the immune response and compromise the body's ability to regulate inflammation adequately. Research is ongoing to elucidate the specific mechanisms underlying cortisol sensitivity in autoimmune hepatitis.

Stress and Disease Flares:

Stress can potentially trigger disease flares or exacerbate symptoms in individuals with autoimmune hepatitis. During times of stress, cortisol levels typically increase as part of the body's stress response. However, in autoimmune hepatitis, the interplay between stress, cortisol levels, and disease activity is complex and may vary among individuals. Some studies suggest that psychological stress may influence disease activity, while others have not found a consistent correlation.

Treatment Considerations:

Cortisol-like medications, such as corticosteroids, are commonly prescribed for autoimmune hepatitis treatment. These medications help suppress the immune response and reduce liver inflammation. By mimicking the effects of cortisol, corticosteroids can help manage symptoms, control disease activity, and prevent disease progression. However, long-term use of corticosteroids may have side effects, necessitating careful monitoring and a gradual tapering of the medication.

Supporting Autoimmune Hepatitis Management:

While the role of cortisol in autoimmune hepatitis is complex and multifaceted, there are strategies to support disease management and overall well-being:

Medication Adherence:

Follow the prescribed treatment plan outlined by your healthcare provider. This may involve taking corticosteroids or other immunosuppressive medications to manage inflammation and prevent disease progression. Adhering to the prescribed medication regimen is crucial for effective disease management.

Regular Monitoring:

Regularly monitor disease activity and liver function through blood tests and imaging studies as recommended by your healthcare provider. These assessments can help gauge treatment response, detect any changes in disease activity, and guide adjustments to the treatment plan if necessary.

Stress Management:

Engage in stress-reducing activities to support overall well-being. Stress management techniques such as relaxation exercises, meditation, engaging in hobbies, and seeking social support can help alleviate stress and potentially influence disease activity. However, it's important to note that stress management alone may not be sufficient to control autoimmune hepatitis, and medical treatment remains essential.

Healthy Lifestyle Choices:

Adopting a healthy lifestyle can contribute to overall well-being and potentially support disease management. This includes maintaining a balanced diet, engaging in regular physical activity (as advised by your healthcare provider), getting sufficient sleep, and avoiding excessive ... consumption. While lifestyle modifications may not directly impact cortisol levels, they can contribute to overall health and potentially influence disease outcomes.

So,

Understanding the intricate relationship between cortisol and autoimmune hepatitis is an ongoing area of research. Cortisol, as a key player in immune regulation and the body's response to stress, exerts influence on the development and progression of autoimmune hepatitis. The interplay between cortisol levels, immune dysregulation, and disease activity in autoimmune hepatitis is complex and multifaceted, requiring further investigation.

In managing autoimmune hepatitis, a comprehensive approach that combines medical treatment, regular monitoring, stress management, and healthy lifestyle choices is crucial. It's important to work closely with healthcare professionals specializing in hepatology and autoimmune diseases to develop an individualized treatment plan and receive ongoing support.

By advancing our knowledge, conducting further research, and promoting a multidisciplinary approach to autoimmune hepatitis management, we can strive to improve patient outcomes, enhance quality of life, and continue making progress in the understanding of this complex autoimmune liver disease.

Please note that this chapter provides insights into the relationship between cortisol and autoimmune hepatitis. However, it should not replace professional medical advice or assessment. If you have specific concerns or questions about your condition, consult with healthcare professionals who can provide personalized guidance based on your unique circumstances.

Chapter 72: Unveiling the Impact of Cortisol on the Body's Response to Psychological Trauma

We will delve into the intricate relationship between cortisol and the body's response to psychological trauma. Psychological trauma, such as experiencing a distressing event or ongoing stress, can have profound effects on our mental and physical well-being. Cortisol, often referred to as the "stress hormone," plays a crucial role in our body's stress response and the regulation of various physiological processes. In this chapter, we will explore how cortisol influences the body's response to psychological trauma, shedding light on the complex interplay between this hormone and our mental and emotional health.

Understanding Psychological Trauma:

Before we dive into the impact of cortisol, let's establish a foundational understanding of psychological trauma. Psychological trauma can occur as a result of experiencing or witnessing a distressing event that overwhelms an individual's ability to cope. This can include events such as accidents, natural disasters, violence, abuse, or ongoing stressors. Trauma can have long-lasting effects on an individual's emotional, cognitive, and physical well-being, affecting various aspects of their life.

The Role of Cortisol in the Stress Response:

Cortisol is a hormone released by the adrenal glands in response to stress. It plays a vital role in our body's stress response, helping to regulate physiological processes and restore balance. When faced with psychological trauma, cortisol levels can fluctuate in the following ways:

Activation of the Stress Response:

Psychological trauma triggers the body's stress response, leading to an increase in cortisol production. This response is designed to mobilize energy, heighten awareness, and prepare the body for potential threats. Elevated cortisol levels during traumatic experiences enable the body to respond effectively to the immediate demands of the situation.

Altered Cortisol Patterns:

Following a traumatic event, cortisol levels may exhibit altered patterns. Some individuals may experience elevated cortisol levels in the immediate aftermath of trauma, while others may exhibit a blunted cortisol response. These patterns can vary depending on factors such as the nature of the trauma, individual differences in stress response, and the presence of other coexisting factors such as pre-existing mental health conditions.

Chronic Stress and Cortisol Dysregulation:

Prolonged exposure to psychological trauma or chronic stress can lead to dysregulation of cortisol levels. In some cases, individuals may experience heightened and prolonged cortisol release, leading to chronic stress-related symptoms. Conversely, others may exhibit lower-than-normal cortisol levels, potentially indicating exhaustion of the stress response system. These dysregulations can contribute to the development of physical and mental health issues.

The Impact of Cortisol on Mental and Emotional Well-being:

Cortisol influences various aspects of mental and emotional well-being in the context of psychological trauma:

Emotional Regulation:

Cortisol plays a role in regulating emotional responses. Elevated cortisol levels during and after a traumatic event can influence emotional reactivity, potentially leading to heightened anxiety, fear, or hyperarousal. On the other hand, dysregulation of cortisol levels may contribute to emotional dysregulation, leading to difficulties in managing emotions or experiencing mood disturbances.

Memory and Cognitive Function:

Cortisol influences memory formation and retrieval. During traumatic experiences, cortisol can modulate memory consolidation, potentially impacting the formation and retrieval of memories related to the traumatic event. Dysregulation of cortisol levels may affect memory processes, contributing to symptoms such as intrusive memories, dissociation, or difficulties in recalling specific details of the traumatic event.

Sleep and Fatigue:

Cortisol levels follow a diurnal pattern, with higher levels in the morning and lower levels in the evening. However, in individuals who have experienced psychological trauma, cortisol dysregulation can disrupt the normal sleep-wake cycle. This can result in sleep disturbances, such as insomnia or nightmares, and increased feelings of fatigue or lethargy.

Coping and Resilience:

Cortisol levels can influence an individual's ability to cope with and recover from traumatic experiences. Adequate cortisol release during and after trauma may support resilience and adaptive coping strategies. Conversely, dysregulated cortisol levels or chronic stress-related cortisol dysregulation may impede the ability to effectively cope with trauma, potentially contributing to the development of post-traumatic stress symptoms.

Supporting Recovery and Resilience:

While the impact of cortisol on the body's response to psychological trauma is complex, there are strategies that can support recovery and foster resilience:

Trauma-Informed Therapies:

Engage in trauma-informed therapies, such as cognitive-behavioral therapy (CBT), eye movement desensitization and reprocessing (EMDR), or trauma-focused therapy. These approaches aim to help individuals process and integrate traumatic experiences, develop healthy coping mechanisms, and regulate emotions effectively.

Social Support and Connection:

Maintain social connections and seek support from trusted individuals. Strong social support networks can provide a sense of belonging, understanding, and validation, which can contribute to emotional well-being and recovery from trauma.

Self-Care and Stress Reduction:

Prioritize self-care practices that promote relaxation, stress reduction, and overall well-being. This can include activities such as mindfulness, meditation, deep breathing exercises, regular physical exercise, engaging in hobbies, and getting sufficient restful sleep. These practices can help regulate cortisol levels and support the body's stress response system.

Professional Support:

If you are experiencing significant distress or struggling to cope with the aftermath of psychological trauma, seek professional help from mental health professionals. They can provide individualized support, assessment, and evidence-based interventions tailored to your unique needs.

So,

Cortisol plays a multifaceted role in the body's response to psychological trauma. It influences the stress response, emotional regulation, memory, sleep patterns, and coping mechanisms. The interplay between cortisol and psychological trauma is complex and varies among individuals. By understanding the impact of cortisol and implementing supportive strategies, individuals can work toward recovery, resilience, and improved well-being in the aftermath of trauma.

It's important to note that this chapter provides insights into the relationship between cortisol and the body's response to psychological trauma. However, it should not replace professional medical or psychological advice. If you have experienced psychological trauma or are struggling with its aftermath, consult with mental health professionals who can provide personalized guidance and support based on your unique circumstances.

Chapter 73: Unveiling the Role of Cortisol in Heart Failure

We will embark on an exploration of the role of cortisol in the development and progression of heart failure. Heart failure is a complex condition characterized by the heart's inability to pump blood effectively, leading to a range of symptoms and complications. Cortisol, often referred to as the "stress hormone," plays a vital role in regulating various physiological processes, including cardiovascular function. In this chapter, we will delve into the influence of cortisol on the development and progression of heart failure, shedding light on the complex interplay between this hormone and cardiovascular health.

Understanding Heart Failure:

Before we delve into the role of cortisol, let's establish a foundational understanding of heart failure. Heart failure occurs when the heart's ability to pump blood is compromised, either due to a weakened heart muscle (systolic heart failure) or impaired relaxation and filling of the heart chambers (diastolic heart failure). Common causes of heart failure include coronary artery disease, high blood pressure, heart valve disorders, and certain medical conditions or lifestyle factors. Heart failure can lead to symptoms such as shortness of breath, fatigue, fluid retention, and reduced exercise tolerance.

The Impact of Cortisol on Heart Failure:

Cortisol, as a key player in the stress response and immune regulation, can influence the development and progression of heart failure in several ways:

Inflammation and Fibrosis:

Cortisol exerts anti-inflammatory effects in the body. In heart failure, chronic inflammation, and excessive fibrosis (scar tissue formation) contribute to the progressive deterioration of the heart muscle. While cortisol can help modulate inflammation, prolonged and excessive cortisol exposure may contribute to an imbalance in the immune response, leading to increased inflammation and fibrosis in the heart muscle.

Sodium and Fluid Balance:

Cortisol affects fluid and electrolyte balance in the body. In heart failure, maintaining proper sodium and fluid balance is crucial to alleviate symptoms and reduce stress on the heart. However, elevated cortisol levels can disrupt this balance by increasing sodium reabsorption in the kidneys and promoting fluid retention. This can exacerbate fluid overload and contribute to the symptoms of heart failure.

Blood Pressure Regulation:

Cortisol influences blood pressure regulation by affecting blood vessel constriction and the function of the renin-angiotensin-aldosterone system. In heart failure, the body's compensatory mechanisms attempt to maintain blood pressure and cardiac output. However, dysregulation of cortisol levels can lead to increased blood pressure, further straining the heart and potentially worsening heart failure symptoms.

Cardiac Remodeling:

Cortisol can influence cardiac remodeling, which refers to the structural and functional changes that occur in the heart in response to injury or chronic stress. In heart failure, chronic exposure to cortisol may contribute to adverse cardiac remodeling, including hypertrophy (enlargement) of the heart muscle and changes in the heart's shape and function. These changes can impair the heart's ability to pump blood efficiently.

Managing Cortisol Levels and Heart Failure:

While the impact of cortisol on heart failure is complex, there are strategies to support heart health and manage cortisol levels:

Medication Adherence:

Follow the prescribed treatment plan outlined by your healthcare provider for heart failure management. Medications such as beta-blockers, angiotensin-converting enzyme (ACE) inhibitors, or angiotensin receptor blockers (ARBs) may be prescribed to help alleviate symptoms, reduce stress on the heart, and improve cardiac function. Adhering to the prescribed medication regimen is crucial for effective heart failure management.

Stress Reduction and Lifestyle Modifications:

Engage in stress-reducing activities and adopt healthy lifestyle choices. Chronic stress can contribute to elevated cortisol levels and may worsen heart failure symptoms. Practicing relaxation techniques, engaging in hobbies, regular physical exercise (as advised by your healthcare provider), getting sufficient sleep, and adopting a heart-healthy diet can help manage stress and support overall heart health.

Weight Management:

Maintain a healthy weight or work towards achieving a healthy weight if overweight or obese. Excess weight can strain the heart and exacerbate heart failure symptoms. A balanced diet, portion control, and regular physical activity, tailored to your individual needs and capabilities, can support weight management and overall heart health.

Regular Monitoring:

Regularly monitor heart failure symptoms, blood pressure, and fluid balance, as recommended by your healthcare provider. This may involve tracking weight, monitoring fluid intake and output, and reporting any changes in symptoms promptly. Regular check-ups and tests can help detect any changes in heart function and guide adjustments to the treatment plan if necessary.

So,

Cortisol, as a hormone involved in the stress response and immune regulation, can influence the development and progression of heart failure. The impact of cortisol on heart failure is complex and multifaceted, involving inflammation, fluid balance, blood pressure regulation, and cardiac remodeling. By managing cortisol levels through stress reduction, lifestyle modifications, and adhering to the prescribed treatment plan, individuals with heart failure can support heart health, alleviate symptoms, and potentially improve overall well-being.

It's important to note that this chapter provides insights into the relationship between cortisol and heart failure. However, it should not replace professional medical advice or assessment. If you have specific concerns or questions about your condition, consult with healthcare professionals who can provide personalized guidance based on your unique circumstances.

Chapter 74: Shedding Light on the Influence of Pesticides and Insecticides on Cortisol Levels

We will delve into the intriguing question of whether cortisol levels can be influenced by exposure to pesticides and insecticides. Pesticides and insecticides are commonly used to control pests and protect crops, but their impact on human health has raised concerns. Cortisol, known as the "stress hormone," plays a vital role in our body's stress response and the regulation of various physiological processes. In this chapter, we will explore the potential influence of pesticides and insecticides on cortisol levels, shedding light on the complex interplay between these chemicals and our hormonal balance.

Understanding Pesticides and Insecticides:

Pesticides and insecticides are chemical substances designed to kill or control pests such as insects, weeds, and fungi. They can be categorized into different classes based on their composition and intended targets. While pesticides and insecticides have proven effective in agricultural and public health settings, there is growing concern about their potential impact on human health due to their widespread use and persistence in the environment.

The Potential Influence of Pesticides and Insecticides on Cortisol Levels:

Emerging research suggests that exposure to certain pesticides and insecticides may have the potential to influence cortisol levels in the following ways:

Disruption of the HPA Axis:

The hypothalamic-pituitary-adrenal (HPA) axis is responsible for regulating cortisol production. Some studies indicate that certain pesticides and insecticides may disrupt the HPA axis, leading to alterations in cortisol production and release. These chemicals can interfere with the normal functioning of the hypothalamus, pituitary gland, or adrenal glands, thereby impacting the regulation of cortisol.

Oxidative Stress and Inflammation:

Exposure to pesticides and insecticides can induce oxidative stress and trigger inflammatory responses in the body. Chronic inflammation and oxidative stress have been associated with dysregulation of cortisol levels. The body's response to the toxic effects of these chemicals may lead to alterations in cortisol production and metabolism, potentially affecting cortisol levels.

Endocrine Disrupting Properties:

Some pesticides and insecticides are known or suspected to have endocrine-disrupting properties. Endocrine disruptors can interfere with the normal function of hormones in the body, including cortisol. They can mimic or block hormone signals, leading to hormonal imbalances. While more research is needed to understand the specific effects of these chemicals on cortisol, their potential to disrupt endocrine function raises concerns.

Individual Variations and Susceptibility:

It's important to note that individual variations in response to pesticides and insecticides may exist. Factors such as genetics, age, underlying health conditions, and duration and intensity of exposure can influence how these chemicals interact with the body's hormonal system, including cortisol regulation. Some individuals may be more susceptible to the effects of pesticides and insecticides on cortisol levels than others.

Mitigating Exposure and Promoting Hormonal Balance:

While the impact of pesticides and insecticides on cortisol levels is still an evolving field of research, there are steps you can take to minimize exposure and promote hormonal balance:

Choose Organic and Locally Sourced Foods:

Opt for organic produce and locally sourced foods whenever possible. Organic farming practices minimize the use of synthetic pesticides and insecticides, reducing the potential exposure to these chemicals. Locally sourced foods also tend to have lower pesticide residue levels.

Wash and Peel Fruits and Vegetables:

Thoroughly wash and, when appropriate, peel fruits and vegetables to reduce pesticide residues. This simple practice can help minimize potential exposure to pesticides and insecticides present on the surface of produce.

Practice Integrated Pest Management:

Support and promote integrated pest management (IPM) practices. IPM focuses on sustainable pest control strategies that minimize the use of chemical pesticides and insecticides. It emphasizes the use of alternative methods such as biological control, crop rotation, and cultural practices to manage pests effectively.

Follow Safety Guidelines:

If you work in agricultural or pest control settings, follow recommended safety guidelines and wear appropriate protective clothing to minimize direct contact with pesticides and insecticides. Proper storage, handling, and disposal of these chemicals are crucial to prevent unnecessary exposure.

Advocate for Responsible Use and Regulations:

Support efforts to enhance regulations and promote responsible use of pesticides and insecticides. Engage in community initiatives and advocate for policies that prioritize human health and environmental sustainability.

So,

While the influence of pesticides and insecticides on cortisol levels is an area of ongoing research, it is essential to remain vigilant about minimizing exposure and promoting hormonal balance. The potential disruption of cortisol regulation by these chemicals raises concerns about their impact on human health. By adopting practices such as choosing organic foods, practicing integrated pest management, following safety guidelines, and advocating for responsible use and regulations, we can take steps to mitigate exposure and promote a healthier environment.

It's important to note that this chapter provides insights into the potential influence of pesticides and insecticides on cortisol levels. However, it should not replace professional advice or assessment. If you have specific concerns about exposure to these chemicals or potential health effects, consult with healthcare professionals or toxicology experts who can provide personalized guidance based on your unique circumstances.

Chapter 75: Unraveling the Impact of Cortisol on the Body's Response to Chemotherapy

We will embark on a journey to explore the intriguing question of how cortisol impacts the body's response to chemotherapy. Chemotherapy is a widely used treatment for cancer that involves the use of powerful medications to destroy cancer cells. Cortisol, known as the "stress hormone," plays a crucial role in our body's stress response and the regulation of various physiological processes. In this chapter, we will delve into the multifaceted interplay between cortisol and chemotherapy, shedding light on its impact on treatment outcomes and the well-being of individuals undergoing chemotherapy.

Understanding Chemotherapy:

Chemotherapy is a systemic treatment that uses medications to target and destroy rapidly dividing cancer cells throughout the body. It is a cornerstone of cancer treatment and can be administered in various ways, including oral pills, intravenous infusion, or injections. Chemotherapy works by interfering with the cancer cells' ability to divide and multiply, thereby halting their growth or causing cell death. While chemotherapy can be effective in combating cancer, it often comes with a range of side effects due to its impact on both cancer and normal cells.

The Role of Cortisol in Chemotherapy:

Cortisol, as a key player in our body's stress response system, can influence the body's response to chemotherapy in several ways:

Immune System Modulation:

Chemotherapy can suppress the immune system, making it challenging for the body to fight infections and recover from treatment. Cortisol, as a natural immune regulator, can impact the immune response during chemotherapy. However, the exact role of cortisol in modulating the immune system during chemotherapy is complex and requires further investigation.

Inflammation and Side Effects:

Chemotherapy can trigger inflammation in the body, leading to side effects such as fatigue, nausea, and pain. Cortisol plays a role in regulating the inflammatory response. Elevated cortisol levels during chemotherapy may help mitigate excessive inflammation and reduce the severity of certain side effects. However, chronic, or prolonged elevation of cortisol may contribute to a range of other adverse effects.

Stress Response and Emotional Well-being:

Undergoing chemotherapy can be physically and emotionally demanding. Cortisol, as the primary hormone involved in the stress response, is intricately linked to emotional well-being and mood regulation. Fluctuations in cortisol levels during chemotherapy may contribute to emotional changes and impact the overall psychological experience of treatment.

Corticosteroids as Adjunct Therapy:

Corticosteroids, synthetic versions of cortisol, are frequently used as adjunct therapy in chemotherapy protocols. These medications help manage side effects such as nausea, allergic reactions, and inflammation. By supplementing cortisol levels in the body, corticosteroids can support treatment tolerability and enhance overall treatment outcomes.

Navigating Cortisol and Chemotherapy:

While the influence of cortisol on chemotherapy outcomes is complex, there are strategies to support individuals undergoing chemotherapy and optimize treatment efficacy:

Emotional Support and Stress Management:

The emotional and psychological well-being of individuals undergoing chemotherapy is paramount. Engage in stress management techniques such as relaxation exercises, mindfulness, and seeking emotional support from loved ones or support groups. These practices can help modulate cortisol levels, improve emotional well-being, and promote resilience during treatment.

Adherence to Treatment Plan:

Strict adherence to the prescribed chemotherapy treatment plan is crucial. Follow the recommended medication schedule, dosage, and any additional therapies such as corticosteroids as advised by your healthcare provider. Consistency in treatment administration is essential for achieving optimal outcomes and managing potential side effects.

Open Communication with Healthcare Team:

Maintain open and honest communication with your healthcare team throughout your chemotherapy journey. They can provide guidance on managing side effects, monitor your well-being, and make necessary adjustments to the treatment plan based on your individual response and needs.

Lifestyle Considerations:

Adopt a healthy lifestyle during chemotherapy. Focus on proper nutrition, hydration, and regular physical activity as recommended by your healthcare provider. These lifestyle choices can support overall well-being, help manage cortisol levels, and enhance treatment tolerance.

So,

The interplay between cortisol and chemotherapy is intricate, and the exact mechanisms underlying their relationship are still being explored. Cortisol, as a key hormone involved in stress response and immune regulation, may influence treatment outcomes, immune response, and emotional well-being during chemotherapy. By prioritizing emotional support, adhering to treatment plans, maintaining open communication with healthcare providers, and adopting a healthy lifestyle, individuals undergoing chemotherapy can optimize their treatment experience and enhance overall well-being.

It's important to note that this chapter provides insights into the potential impact of cortisol on the body's response to chemotherapy. However, it should not replace professional medical advice or assessment. If you have specific concerns or questions about your chemotherapy treatment, consult with your healthcare provider, who can provide personalized guidance based on your unique circumstances.

Chapter 76: Navigating the Impact of Cortisol on the Body's Response to Hormonal Changes During Puberty

We will embark on an exploration of how cortisol influences the body's response to the hormonal changes that occur during puberty. Puberty is a transformative phase in an individual's life, marked by significant physical, emotional, and hormonal changes. Cortisol, known as the "stress hormone," plays a crucial role in our body's stress response and the regulation of various physiological processes. In this chapter, we will delve into the intricate interplay between cortisol and the hormonal changes that unfold during puberty, shedding light on its impact on growth, development, and emotional well-being.

Understanding Puberty and Hormonal Changes:

Puberty is a period of maturation during which the body undergoes significant changes to reach reproductive maturity. It is characterized by the activation of the hypothalamic-pituitary-gonadal (HPG) axis, which stimulates the production of sex hormones such as estrogen and testosterone. These hormones play a central role in the development of secondary sexual characteristics, the maturation of reproductive organs, and the initiation of the menstrual cycle in females and sperm production in males.

The Role of Cortisol in Puberty:

Cortisol, as a key player in our body's stress response system, can influence the body's response to the hormonal changes of puberty in several ways:

Impact on Growth and Development:

Cortisol plays a role in regulating growth and development during puberty. It interacts with growth hormone (GH) and insulin-like growth factor 1 (IGF-1), two hormones involved in skeletal growth and body composition. Elevated cortisol levels may affect the balance between GH and IGF-1, potentially influencing growth patterns and body composition during this critical period.

Emotional and Behavioral Effects:

Puberty is often accompanied by emotional and behavioral changes due to the complex interplay between hormones and brain development. Cortisol, as a hormone involved in stress response, can impact emotional well-being and mood regulation during this sensitive phase. Fluctuations in cortisol levels may contribute to mood swings, emotional sensitivity, and stress-related behaviors.

Influence on the Hypothalamic-Pituitary-Gonadal (HPG) Axis:

Cortisol can modulate the HPG axis, which regulates the production of sex hormones during puberty. Stressful experiences and elevated cortisol levels may disrupt the delicate balance of the HPG axis, potentially affecting the timing and progression of puberty. The impact of cortisol on the HPG axis may vary among individuals, influenced by genetic and environmental factors.

Interplay with Other Hormones:

Puberty involves a complex interplay of various hormones, including cortisol, sex hormones, and thyroid hormones. Cortisol can interact with these hormones, influencing their production, release, and overall effects on the body. The intricate hormonal web during puberty underscores the need for a delicate balance to ensure healthy growth and development.

Navigating Cortisol and Puberty:

While the influence of cortisol on puberty is complex and multifaceted, there are strategies to support individuals during this transformative phase:

Stress Management:

Promote stress management techniques that can help modulate cortisol levels and support emotional well-being. Engage in activities such as exercise, mindfulness, deep breathing, and engaging in hobbies or creative outlets. These practices can help reduce stress and enhance resilience during this period of hormonal changes.

Healthy Lifestyle Choices:

Encourage healthy lifestyle choices that promote overall well-being. Focus on proper nutrition, regular physical activity, and sufficient sleep. A balanced and nutritious diet, combined with regular exercise, can contribute to hormonal balance, and support healthy growth and development.

Open Communication:

Maintain open and supportive communication with adolescents going through puberty. Encourage them to express their feelings and concerns, providing a safe space for discussing the physical and emotional changes they are experiencing. Supportive relationships and open dialogue can help adolescents navigate the challenges of puberty and reduce stress levels.

Seeking Professional Guidance:

If significant emotional or behavioral concerns arise during puberty, consider seeking guidance from healthcare professionals or mental health experts. They can provide personalized support, address specific challenges, and offer strategies to manage stress and promote well-being.

So,

The interplay between cortisol and the hormonal change during puberty is intricate and requires a holistic approach to support adolescents during this transformative phase. While cortisol's impact on puberty is still being explored, understanding the potential influence of stress and cortisol on growth, emotional well-being, and hormonal balance can guide strategies to promote a healthy transition into adulthood. By emphasizing stress management, healthy lifestyle choices, open communication, and seeking professional guidance when needed, we can help adolescents navigate puberty with resilience, confidence, and optimal well-being.

It's important to note that this chapter provides insights into the potential impact of cortisol on the body's response to hormonal changes during puberty. However, it should not replace professional medical or psychological advice. If you have specific concerns or questions about your child's puberty or well-being, consult with healthcare providers or experts who can provide personalized guidance based on your unique circumstances.

Chapter 77: Understanding the Role of Cortisol in the Development and Progression of Rheumatoid Arthritis

We will dive into the intriguing question of whether cortisol plays a role in the development and progression of rheumatoid arthritis (RA). Rheumatoid arthritis is a chronic autoimmune disease characterized by joint inflammation, pain, and stiffness. Cortisol, known as the "stress hormone," is a key player in our body's stress response and the regulation of various physiological processes. In this chapter, we will explore the complex interplay between cortisol and RA, shedding light on its potential impact on the disease's onset, progression, and management.

Understanding Rheumatoid Arthritis:

Rheumatoid arthritis is an autoimmune disease that primarily affects the joints. In this condition, the body's immune system mistakenly attacks the synovium, a thin membrane that lines the joints, causing inflammation, pain, and eventual joint damage. The exact cause of RA is still unknown, but it is believed to involve a combination of genetic, environmental, and hormonal factors.

The Role of Cortisol in Rheumatoid Arthritis:

Cortisol, as a key hormone involved in the stress response, can influence the development and progression of RA through various mechanisms:

Immune System Modulation:

Cortisol is known to have immunosuppressive effects, meaning it can suppress the immune system's activity. In the context of RA, this immunosuppressive property may help reduce the excessive immune response responsible for joint inflammation. However, prolonged, or chronic elevation of cortisol levels can weaken the immune system, potentially leading to increased susceptibility to infections and other complications.

Inflammation and Disease Activity:

Inflammation plays a central role in the development and progression of RA. Cortisol can modulate the body's inflammatory response, helping to manage inflammation and reduce disease activity. However, the relationship between cortisol and inflammation in RA is complex, and imbalances in cortisol levels or dysfunction in the body's stress response system may contribute to ongoing inflammation and disease flare-ups.

Stress and Flare-ups:

Stress is known to exacerbate the symptoms of many chronic conditions, including RA. Stressful events or chronic stress can trigger the release of cortisol, which, in turn, can influence the body's inflammatory response and potentially contribute to RA flare-ups. Effective stress management techniques may help individuals with RA better cope with the challenges of the disease and reduce the impact of cortisol-induced flare-ups.

Glucocorticoid Therapy:

Glucocorticoids, synthetic versions of cortisol, are commonly prescribed in RA treatment. These medications have potent anti-inflammatory effects and can help manage symptoms and control disease activity. However, long-term use of glucocorticoids may be associated with side effects, including bone loss, weight gain, and increased risk of infections. Balancing the benefits and risks of glucocorticoid therapy is crucial in the management of RA.

Navigating Cortisol and Rheumatoid Arthritis:

While the influence of cortisol on the development and progression of RA is complex, several strategies can support individuals with RA in managing their condition:

Medication and Treatment:

Work closely with a healthcare team to develop an individualized treatment plan. This plan may include disease-modifying antirheumatic drugs (DMARDs), which target the underlying autoimmune response, and may also involve short-term use of glucocorticoids to manage acute symptoms. Regular monitoring and adjustment of medications based on disease activity and individual response are essential.

Stress Management:

Implement effective stress management techniques to reduce the impact of stress on RA symptoms. Engage in activities such as relaxation exercises, mindfulness, meditation, and engaging in hobbies or activities that promote well-being. These practices can help modulate cortisol levels, reduce stress, and promote overall physical and emotional well-being.

Healthy Lifestyle Choices:

Adopt a healthy lifestyle that includes regular exercise, a balanced diet, and sufficient sleep. Regular physical activity can help improve joint function, reduce pain, and enhance overall well-being. A nutritious diet rich in anti-inflammatory foods, such as fruits, vegetables, and omega-3 fatty acids, may also support joint health and reduce inflammation.

Supportive Therapies:

Explore complementary and alternative therapies such as acupuncture, massage, and physical therapy. These therapies can help alleviate pain, improve joint mobility, and enhance overall quality of life. However, it's important to discuss these options with your healthcare provider to ensure their safety and effectiveness in the context of your RA management.

So,

While the exact role of cortisol in the development and progression of rheumatoid arthritis is still being explored, understanding its potential impact can offer insights into the management and treatment of this chronic autoimmune condition. Cortisol's influence on immune response, inflammation, and stress underscores the importance of a holistic approach that encompasses medication, stress management, healthy lifestyle choices, and supportive therapies. By working closely with healthcare providers, implementing effective stress management techniques, and adopting a healthy lifestyle, individuals with RA can optimize their overall well-being and enhance their ability to manage the challenges associated with the disease.

It's important to note that this chapter provides insights into the potential impact of cortisol on rheumatoid arthritis. However, it should not replace professional medical advice or assessment. If you have specific concerns or questions about your RA management, consult with your healthcare provider, who can provide personalized guidance based on your unique circumstances.

Chapter 78: Understanding the Potential Influence of Electromagnetic Radiation on Cortisol Levels

We will delve into the intriguing question of whether cortisol levels can be influenced by exposure to electromagnetic radiation. Electromagnetic radiation is a form of energy that surrounds us in various forms, such as radio waves, microwaves, visible light, and X-rays. Cortisol, commonly known as the "stress hormone," plays a vital role in our body's stress response and the regulation of various physiological processes. In this chapter, we will explore the existing research and evidence to shed light on the potential relationship between electromagnetic radiation and cortisol levels.

Understanding Electromagnetic Radiation:

Electromagnetic radiation exists in a broad spectrum, ranging from low-frequency waves, such as radio waves, to high-frequency waves, such as X-rays and gamma rays. We encounter electromagnetic radiation from numerous sources in our daily lives, including electronic devices, Wi-Fi signals, power lines, and even natural sources like the sun. The impact of electromagnetic radiation on our health has been a subject of scientific investigation and public interest.

Cortisol and the Stress Response:

Cortisol is a hormone produced by the adrenal glands in response to stress. It helps regulate various physiological processes, including metabolism, immune function, inflammation, and the body's response to stress. Cortisol levels naturally fluctuate throughout the day, following a diurnal pattern with higher levels in the morning and lower levels in the evening. However, chronic, or excessive cortisol elevation can have negative effects on health, including immune suppression, metabolic imbalances, and increased risk of certain diseases.

Exploring the Potential Influence of Electromagnetic Radiation on Cortisol Levels:

The relationship between electromagnetic radiation and cortisol levels is a topic of ongoing scientific investigation. While research in this area is still emerging, some studies suggest a potential connection:

Mobile Phone Radiation:

Several studies have investigated the impact of mobile phone radiation on cortisol levels. Some studies have reported an association between mobile phone use and altered cortisol patterns, including elevated cortisol levels, or disrupted diurnal rhythms. However, other studies have not found significant effects. Further research is needed to clarify these findings and determine the potential mechanisms involved.

Wi-Fi and Electromagnetic Fields (EMFs):

The influence of Wi-Fi and other electromagnetic fields (EMFs) on cortisol levels is still a subject of scientific debate. Some studies have reported changes in cortisol levels in response to exposure to Wi-Fi signals or EMFs from other sources, while others have not found significant effects. The variations in study design, exposure levels, and participant characteristics contribute to the complexity of interpreting the results.

Magnetic Fields and Power Lines:

Exposure to magnetic fields from power lines has also been investigated in relation to cortisol levels. Some studies have suggested a potential association between chronic exposure to magnetic fields and alterations in cortisol levels. However, more research is needed to better understand the mechanisms involved and establish consistent findings.

Individual Variability and Context:

It's important to recognize that individuals may respond differently to electromagnetic radiation based on various factors, including genetic predisposition, existing health conditions, and personal sensitivity. Additionally, the context and duration of exposure may also influence the potential impact on cortisol levels. Further research is necessary to explore these factors and elucidate the potential mechanisms involved.

Practical Considerations and Recommendations:

While the relationship between electromagnetic radiation and cortisol levels is still not fully understood, some practical considerations can help minimize potential risks:

Awareness and Moderation:

Be aware of your exposure to electromagnetic radiation and use electronic devices moderately and purposefully. Minimize unnecessary exposure by keeping devices away from the body when not in use, using speakerphone or hands-free options, and maintaining distance from strong electromagnetic sources.

Create a Low-EMF Environment:

Consider implementing measures to reduce electromagnetic radiation exposure in your immediate environment. This may include using wired connections instead of Wi-Fi when possible, keeping electronic devices at a distance while sleeping, and creating technology-free zones in your home.

Stress Management:

Focus on stress management techniques to support overall well-being. Engage in activities such as exercise, mindfulness, meditation, and relaxation exercises. These practices can help modulate cortisol levels and enhance resilience to various stressors, including electromagnetic radiation.

Stay Informed:

Keep up to date with scientific research and recommendations regarding electromagnetic radiation. The field of study is evolving, and new findings may emerge that provide further insights into the potential impact of electromagnetic radiation on cortisol levels and overall health.

So,

While the influence of electromagnetic radiation on cortisol levels is a topic of ongoing research, it is important to approach the subject with scientific scrutiny and an awareness of the current evidence. While some studies suggest a potential relationship between electromagnetic radiation and cortisol, inconsistencies in the findings and individual variability highlight the need for further investigation. By maintaining a balanced approach, being mindful of exposure, practicing stress management techniques, and staying informed, individuals can take steps to support their well-being in the context of modern technology. It's essential to note that this chapter provides insights into the potential influence of electromagnetic radiation on cortisol levels. However, it should not replace professional medical advice or assessment. If you have specific concerns about electromagnetic radiation or its potential impact on your health, consult with healthcare professionals or experts who can provide personalized guidance based on your unique circumstances.

Chapter 79: Unraveling the Relationship Between Cortisol and the Body's Response to Chronic Fatigue Syndrome

We will delve into the fascinating topic of the relationship between cortisol and the body's response to chronic fatigue syndrome (CFS). Chronic fatigue syndrome, also known as myalgic encephalomyelitis (ME), is a complex and debilitating condition characterized by profound fatigue, along with other symptoms such as impaired cognitive function, unrefreshing sleep, and post-exertional malaise. Cortisol, the "stress hormone," plays a crucial role in regulating our body's stress response and maintaining overall homeostasis. In this chapter, we will explore the intricate interplay between cortisol and CFS, shedding light on its potential influence on the condition's onset, symptoms, and management.

Understanding Chronic Fatigue Syndrome:

Chronic fatigue syndrome is a multifaceted disorder that often presents with a combination of symptoms, making diagnosis challenging. The exact cause of CFS remains unknown, and it is believed to involve a complex interplay of factors, including genetic predisposition, viral infections, immune system dysfunction, and environmental triggers. The condition affects individuals differently, and its impact can range from mild to severe, significantly impairing quality of life.

The Role of Cortisol in Chronic Fatigue Syndrome:

Cortisol, as a key hormone involved in the stress response, may play a role in the manifestation and progression of chronic fatigue syndrome. Here are some aspects to consider:

HPA Axis Dysregulation:

The hypothalamic-pituitary-adrenal (HPA) axis, a complex system involving the hypothalamus, pituitary gland, and adrenal glands, regulates the body's response to stress and influences cortisol production. In CFS, there is evidence of dysregulation in the HPA axis, leading to abnormal cortisol levels and disrupted stress response. Some studies have reported reduced cortisol levels, while others have observed blunted cortisol awakening response or altered diurnal cortisol patterns. These variations may contribute to the fatigue and other symptoms experienced by individuals with CFS.

Impact on Energy Regulation:

Cortisol plays a role in energy metabolism, helping regulate glucose production and utilization. In individuals with CFS, abnormalities in cortisol levels and HPA axis function may impact energy regulation, leading to fatigue and reduced stamina. Dysregulated cortisol levels can influence energy availability, affecting physical and mental function, and exacerbating the symptoms of CFS.

Immune System Dysfunction:

The immune system is closely intertwined with both cortisol and CFS. Cortisol has immunosuppressive effects, helping to dampen inflammation and regulate immune responses. In CFS, immune system dysfunction is often observed, including alterations in cytokine levels and impaired immune response. Dysregulated cortisol levels may contribute to immune dysregulation, potentially exacerbating inflammation, and other immune-related symptoms in individuals with CFS.

Stress Response and Symptom Exacerbation:

Stress, both physical and psychological, can trigger or worsen symptoms in individuals with CFS. The release of cortisol during stress is a vital part of the body's adaptive response. However, in CFS, the stress response may be dysregulated, leading to an abnormal cortisol response and potentially exacerbating symptoms. It is important to note that individuals with CFS may be more sensitive to stressors, including emotional stress, physical exertion, and environmental factors, which can further impact cortisol levels and symptom severity.

Navigating Cortisol and Chronic Fatigue Syndrome:

While the exact relationship between cortisol and chronic fatigue syndrome is complex and multifaceted, several strategies can support individuals with CFS in managing their condition:

Individualized Treatment Approach:

Work closely with a healthcare team experienced in CFS management to develop an individualized treatment plan. This may involve a combination of symptom management strategies, lifestyle adjustments, and targeted interventions to address cortisol dysregulation and other underlying factors contributing to CFS symptoms.

Stress Management Techniques:

Implement stress management techniques to minimize the impact of stress on CFS symptoms. This may include relaxation exercises, mindfulness meditation, pacing activities, and maintaining a balanced lifestyle. By reducing stress and supporting overall well-being, individuals with CFS may experience improved symptom management and enhanced quality of life.

Sleep Hygiene:

Optimize sleep hygiene practices to improve sleep quality and quantity. Establish a regular sleep schedule, create a conducive sleep environment, and implement relaxation techniques before bedtime. Good sleep hygiene can help regulate cortisol levels and promote restorative sleep, which is essential for individuals with CFS.

Graduated Exercise and Activity Management:

Physical activity management is crucial in CFS management. Gradually increasing activity levels based on individual capacity and avoiding overexertion can help manage symptoms and prevent post-exertional malaise. Working with a healthcare provider or physical therapist experienced in CFS management is essential to develop an appropriate exercise program tailored to individual needs.

So,

Understanding the relationship between cortisol and chronic fatigue syndrome offers insights into the complex nature of this condition. Dysregulation in the HPA axis, abnormalities in cortisol levels, and the impact on energy regulation and the immune system may contribute to the development and progression of CFS symptoms. By working closely with healthcare providers, implementing stress management techniques, prioritizing sleep hygiene, and gradually increasing activity levels, individuals with CFS can optimize symptom management and enhance their overall well-being.

It's important to note that this chapter provides insights into the potential relationship between cortisol and chronic fatigue syndrome. However, it should not replace professional medical advice or assessment. If you have specific concerns or questions about your CFS management, consult with your healthcare provider, who can provide personalized guidance based on your unique circumstances.

Chapter 80: Unraveling the Impact of Cortisol on the Body's Response to Chronic Pain Conditions

We will explore the intriguing relationship between cortisol and the body's response to chronic pain conditions. Chronic pain is a complex and challenging condition that affects millions of people worldwide, significantly impacting their quality of life. Cortisol, commonly known as the "stress hormone," plays a crucial role in our body's stress response and the regulation of various physiological processes. In this chapter, we will delve into the multifaceted effects of cortisol on chronic pain, examining its role in pain modulation, inflammation, and the body's response to stress.

Understanding Chronic Pain:

Chronic pain is characterized by persistent or recurrent pain that lasts for longer than three months, often resulting from injury, medical conditions, or neurological disorders. It can manifest in various forms, including musculoskeletal pain, neuropathic pain, and fibromyalgia. Chronic pain not only affects physical well-being but also impacts emotional and psychological aspects of a person's life, leading to decreased mobility, sleep disturbances, and reduced overall quality of life.

The Role of Cortisol in Chronic Pain:

Cortisol, as a key hormone involved in the stress response, can influence the body's perception and response to chronic pain. Here are some important aspects to consider:

Pain Modulation:

Cortisol has the potential to modulate the perception of pain. In situations of acute pain, cortisol levels often rise as part of the body's natural stress response, which may help suppress pain signals and provide temporary pain relief. However, in chronic pain conditions, prolonged cortisol elevation and dysregulation can contribute to a state of heightened pain sensitivity. Chronic stress and persistently high cortisol levels can sensitize pain receptors, leading to increased pain perception and decreased pain tolerance.

Inflammation and Immune Response:

Inflammation plays a significant role in many chronic pain conditions. Cortisol, with its anti-inflammatory properties, helps regulate the body's immune response and dampen inflammation. However, prolonged exposure to stress and chronic elevation of cortisol levels can impair the immune system and lead to a dysregulated inflammatory response. In this state, cortisol's anti-inflammatory effects may be compromised, potentially contributing to increased inflammation and exacerbation of pain in chronic pain conditions.

Stress and Pain Sensitization:

Stress can have a profound impact on pain perception and the body's response to pain. When we experience stress, cortisol levels rise to help the body cope with the stressor. However, chronic stress and ongoing cortisol elevation can sensitize the nervous system, amplifying pain signals and increasing pain sensitivity. Additionally, stress can trigger muscle tension and contribute to the development of myofascial pain syndrome and tension-related pain conditions.

Psychological and Emotional Factors:

The relationship between cortisol and chronic pain is influenced by psychological and emotional factors. Chronic pain often coexists with conditions such as anxiety, depression, and stress-related disorders. These psychological factors can impact cortisol regulation and contribute to altered pain perception and the maintenance of chronic pain states. Furthermore, the stress and emotional burden associated with chronic pain can perpetuate a cycle of elevated cortisol levels, exacerbating pain and leading to a negative impact on mental well-being.

Navigating Cortisol and Chronic Pain:

Managing cortisol levels and its impact on chronic pain requires a comprehensive approach. Here are some strategies to consider:

Stress Management:

Implement stress management techniques to help regulate cortisol levels and reduce the impact of stress on chronic pain. These may include relaxation exercises, mindfulness meditation, deep breathing exercises, and engaging in activities that promote a sense of calm and well-being. By managing stress, individuals can potentially alleviate pain perception and enhance overall well-being.

Physical Activity and Exercise:

Regular physical activity and exercise, tailored to individual capabilities, can have positive effects on cortisol regulation and chronic pain management. Exercise promotes the release of endorphins, the body's natural pain-relieving chemicals, and can help regulate cortisol levels. Engaging in low-impact exercises, such as walking, swimming, or yoga, can provide pain relief, improve mood, and enhance overall physical and mental well-being.

Sleep Hygiene:

Optimize sleep quality and quantity as disrupted sleep can contribute to increased pain perception and cortisol dysregulation. Establish a consistent sleep routine, create a comfortable sleep environment, and practice good sleep hygiene habits. Adequate restful sleep supports cortisol regulation, aids in pain management, and promotes healing.

Holistic Approaches:

Explore complementary and alternative therapies that focus on stress reduction and pain management. Techniques such as acupuncture, massage therapy, mindfulness-based stress reduction, and cognitive-behavioral therapy (CBT) can help address both the physiological and psychological aspects of chronic pain. These approaches aim to reduce cortisol levels, improve pain coping strategies, and enhance overall well-being.

So,

Understanding the impact of cortisol on chronic pain provides valuable insights into the complexity of managing chronic pain conditions. Cortisol's influence on pain modulation, inflammation, stress response, and psychological factors highlights the need for a comprehensive approach to pain management that considers both the physiological and emotional aspects of chronic pain. By implementing stress management techniques, engaging in regular physical activity, optimizing sleep, and exploring holistic approaches, individuals with chronic pain can potentially reduce pain perception, improve function, and enhance their overall quality of life.

It's important to note that this chapter provides insights into the potential relationship between cortisol and chronic pain conditions. However, it should not replace professional medical advice or assessment. If you have specific concerns or questions about your chronic pain management, consult with your healthcare provider, who can provide personalized guidance based on your unique circumstances.

Chapter 81: Unraveling the Role of Cortisol in the Development and Progression of Multiple Sclerosis

We will explore the intriguing relationship between cortisol and the development and progression of multiple sclerosis (MS). Multiple sclerosis is a chronic autoimmune disease that affects the central nervous system, leading to inflammation, demyelination, and neurological dysfunction. Cortisol, commonly known as the "stress hormone," plays a vital role in the body's stress response and has complex interactions with the immune system. In this chapter, we will delve into the multifaceted effects of cortisol on MS, examining its potential role in disease onset, symptom exacerbation, and the overall management of this condition.

Understanding Multiple Sclerosis:

Multiple sclerosis is a complex and unpredictable disease characterized by the immune system's attack on the protective myelin sheath that surrounds nerve fibers in the central nervous system. This attack disrupts the normal transmission of nerve impulses, leading to a wide range of symptoms, including fatigue, muscle weakness, coordination difficulties, and cognitive impairments. The exact cause of MS remains unknown, but it is believed to involve a combination of genetic predisposition, environmental factors, and an abnormal immune response.

The Role of Cortisol in Multiple Sclerosis:

Cortisol, as a key hormone involved in the stress response, can impact various aspects of multiple sclerosis. Here are some important considerations:

Immune Modulation:

Cortisol has immunomodulatory effects, meaning it helps regulate the immune system's response to various stimuli. In the context of multiple sclerosis, dysregulation in the immune system plays a critical role in the disease's pathogenesis. Cortisol has the potential to suppress inflammatory responses and dampen immune activity.

However, in MS, the balance between cortisol's immunosuppressive effects and the dysregulated immune response is complex and not fully understood. The interplay between cortisol and the immune system in MS is a topic of ongoing research.

Impact on Symptom Exacerbation:

Stress and cortisol levels have been linked to symptom exacerbation in multiple sclerosis. Stress, whether physical or psychological, can trigger immune system responses and potentially worsen MS symptoms. Cortisol, released during stress, may have a modulatory effect on the immune response, which could influence the severity and duration of MS relapses. However, it's important to note that stress alone is not the sole determinant of MS relapses, as the disease course is multifactorial and varies among individuals.

Impact on Quality of Life:

Cortisol and its relationship with stress can significantly affect the quality of life of individuals living with multiple sclerosis. The emotional and psychological toll of managing a chronic disease like MS can lead to increased stress levels, potentially impacting cortisol regulation. The resulting cortisol dysregulation may contribute to the development or worsening of secondary symptoms such as fatigue, sleep disturbances, and mood changes. Managing stress and optimizing cortisol regulation can positively impact overall well-being and improve the management of MS symptoms.

Treatment Considerations:

Cortisol and its interactions with the immune system have implications for MS treatment strategies. Some disease-modifying therapies used in MS management aim to modulate immune responses and reduce inflammation. Understanding how these therapies impact cortisol regulation is important for optimizing treatment outcomes and minimizing potential side effects related to cortisol dysregulation.

Navigating Cortisol and Multiple Sclerosis:

Managing cortisol levels and its impact on multiple sclerosis requires a comprehensive approach. Here are some strategies to consider:

Stress Management:

Implement stress management techniques to help regulate cortisol levels and minimize stress-related exacerbation of MS symptoms. This may include relaxation exercises, mindfulness meditation, engaging in hobbies, seeking social support, and maintaining a balanced lifestyle. By managing stress, individuals with MS can potentially improve symptom management and enhance overall well-being.

Exercise and Physical Activity:

Engage in regular physical activity and exercise, tailored to individual capabilities, and guided by healthcare professionals. Exercise has been shown to have positive effects on cortisol regulation, mood, and overall physical well-being. It can also help improve fatigue, strength, and balance, which are common concerns in individuals with MS.

Supportive Therapies:

Complementary and alternative therapies such as yoga, acupuncture, and massage therapy may provide additional support for managing stress, improving relaxation, and enhancing overall well-being. These therapies can be valuable additions to conventional treatments and should be discussed with healthcare providers to ensure safety and appropriateness for individual.

Chapter 82: Unraveling the Influence of Industrial Chemicals and Solvents on Cortisol Levels

We will explore the fascinating relationship between exposure to industrial chemicals and solvents and their potential influence on cortisol levels. In today's industrialized world, we are exposed to a variety of chemicals and solvents in our daily lives, ranging from cleaning products and paints to manufacturing and industrial processes. Cortisol, often referred to as the "stress hormone," plays a crucial role in the body's stress response and the regulation of various physiological processes. In this chapter, we will delve into the potential effects of industrial chemicals and solvents on cortisol levels, examining the possible mechanisms of influence and the implications for human health.

Understanding Industrial Chemicals and Solvents:

Industrial chemicals and solvents are substances used in various industrial processes, manufacturing, cleaning, and maintenance activities. They encompass a wide range of compounds, including volatile organic compounds (VOCs), heavy metals, pesticides, and industrial byproducts. These substances can enter the body through inhalation, ingestion, or skin contact and have the potential to interact with various biological systems.

Cortisol and the Stress Response:

Cortisol is a hormone produced by the adrenal glands in response to stress. It plays a vital role in the body's stress response by regulating metabolism, immune function, and inflammation. Cortisol levels typically fluctuate throughout the day, following a diurnal pattern with higher levels in the morning and lower levels in the evening. However, chronic exposure to stressors, including chemical and environmental factors, can disrupt this natural cortisol rhythm and have implications for health.

The Influence of Industrial Chemicals and Solvents on Cortisol Levels:

Exposure to industrial chemicals and solvents can potentially affect cortisol levels through several mechanisms. Here are some important considerations:

Endocrine Disruption:

Certain industrial chemicals and solvents have been identified as endocrine disruptors, meaning they can interfere with the normal functioning of the endocrine system, including the regulation of hormones like cortisol. These substances can mimic or interfere with hormone signaling, leading to alterations in hormone production, metabolism, or clearance. As a result, cortisol regulation may be disrupted, potentially leading to abnormal cortisol levels.

Oxidative Stress and Inflammation:

Industrial chemicals and solvents can induce oxidative stress and inflammation in the body. Oxidative stress occurs when there is an imbalance between the production of reactive oxygen species (ROS) and the body's antioxidant defenses. This imbalance can trigger inflammatory responses and cellular damage. Chronic exposure to oxidative stress and inflammation can disrupt cortisol regulation, leading to dysregulation of the stress response.

Neurological Effects:

Some industrial chemicals and solvents can cross the blood-brain barrier and directly affect the central nervous system. These substances may impact brain structures involved in the regulation of cortisol, such as the hypothalamus and the pituitary gland. Disruption of these brain regions can lead to abnormalities in cortisol synthesis, secretion, or feedback regulation, potentially altering cortisol levels.

Liver Function:

The liver plays a crucial role in the metabolism and clearance of hormones, including cortisol. Exposure to certain industrial chemicals and solvents can impair liver function, affecting the metabolism and elimination of cortisol from the body. This can result in altered cortisol levels and potential dysregulation of the stress response.

Navigating Industrial Chemicals, Solvents, and Cortisol Levels:

Minimizing exposure to industrial chemicals and solvents and promoting a healthy environment is essential for maintaining cortisol levels within a balanced range. Here are some strategies to consider:

Awareness and Education:

Educate yourself about the potential sources of industrial chemicals and solvents in your environment. Stay informed about workplace safety guidelines, proper handling procedures, and protective measures to reduce exposure risks. Understanding potential hazards and taking appropriate precautions can help minimize the impact on cortisol levels and overall health.

Protective Measures:

When working with or around industrial chemicals and solvents, follow recommended safety practices, such as using personal protective equipment (PPE) and ensuring proper ventilation in workspaces. These measures can help reduce the likelihood of direct exposure and limit the potential impact on cortisol regulation.

Environmental Considerations:

Be mindful of the products and materials you use in your daily life. Opt for environmentally friendly and non-toxic alternatives whenever possible. Choose cleaning products, paints, and household items that have low chemical emissions and are labeled as "VOC-free" or "low VOC." By reducing exposure to harmful chemicals, you can promote a healthier living environment and potentially support balanced cortisol levels.

Detoxification Support:

Supporting your body's natural detoxification processes can aid in minimizing the adverse effects of industrial chemicals and solvents. Focus on a nutrient-rich diet that includes foods with liver-supporting properties, such as cruciferous vegetables, turmeric, and green tea. Stay hydrated, engage in regular exercise, and consider consulting with a healthcare professional about specific detoxification protocols if necessary.

So,

Understanding the potential influence of industrial chemicals and solvents on cortisol levels provides valuable insights into the complex interplay between environmental factors and human health. While it is challenging to completely avoid exposure to these substances, adopting strategies to minimize exposure and promote a healthy environment can help maintain balanced cortisol levels. By being mindful of potential sources of exposure, taking protective measures, and supporting the body's natural detoxification processes, individuals can reduce the potential impact on cortisol regulation and promote overall well-being.

It's important to note that this chapter provides insights into the potential relationship between industrial chemicals, solvents, and cortisol levels. However, it should not replace professional medical advice or assessment. If you have specific concerns about exposure to industrial chemicals and solvents or potential health effects, consult with a healthcare professional or occupational health specialist who can provide personalized guidance based on your unique circumstances.

Chapter 83: Unveiling the Impact of Cortisol on the Body's Response to Organ Transplantation

We will delve into the intriguing relationship between cortisol and the body's response to organ transplantation. Organ transplantation is a life-saving procedure that involves replacing a damaged or non-functioning organ with a healthy organ from a donor. Cortisol, commonly known as the "stress hormone," plays a vital role in the body's stress response and has complex interactions with the immune system. In this chapter, we will explore the multifaceted effects of cortisol on organ transplantation, examining its influence on transplant outcomes, rejection, and the management of immunosuppression.

Understanding Organ Transplantation:

Organ transplantation is a medical procedure performed to replace a failed or diseased organ with a healthy one from a living or deceased donor. This procedure offers a lifeline to individuals suffering from end-stage organ failure, providing them with a chance to regain their health and improve their quality of life. Transplantation can involve various organs such as the heart, liver, kidneys, lungs, and pancreas, each with its unique considerations and challenges.

The Role of Cortisol in Organ Transplantation:

Cortisol, as a key hormone involved in the stress response, can impact various aspects of organ transplantation. Here are some important considerations:

Transplant Outcome:

Cortisol levels before and after transplantation can influence the overall outcome of the procedure. Higher pre-transplant cortisol levels have been associated with an increased risk of complications and worse outcomes following transplantation. High levels of cortisol can disrupt the delicate balance between the immune system and the transplanted organ, potentially leading to increased inflammation, impaired wound healing, and higher rates of infection.

Immune Response and Rejection:

The immune system plays a crucial role in the success or failure of organ transplantation. Cortisol has immunomodulatory effects, meaning it can modulate the immune response. In the context of organ transplantation, the goal is to suppress the immune system to prevent rejection of the transplanted organ. Corticosteroids, synthetic versions of cortisol, are commonly used as immunosuppressive agents to prevent rejection. They work by suppressing the immune system's inflammatory response, reducing the risk of rejection. However, finding the right balance is essential, as excessive immunosuppression can increase the risk of infection, while insufficient suppression may lead to rejection.

Steroid-Based Immunosuppression:

Corticosteroids, such as prednisone and methylprednisolone, are often part of the immunosuppressive regimen following organ transplantation. These medications mimic the actions of cortisol and help prevent rejection by suppressing the immune response. However, long-term use of corticosteroids can have side effects, including weight gain, bone loss, high blood pressure, and increased susceptibility to infections. Finding the optimal dosage and duration of corticosteroid therapy is crucial to balance the need for immunosuppression and minimize the risk of complications.

Stress and Cortisol Dysregulation:

Organ transplantation is a major life event that can induce significant physical and emotional stress for both the transplant recipient and the donor. This stress can lead to cortisol dysregulation, with potential implications for the immune response and overall transplant outcomes. Elevated stress and cortisol levels can contribute to increased inflammation, delayed wound healing, and impaired recovery. Therefore, managing stress and promoting psychological well-being before and after transplantation is important to optimize outcomes.

Navigating Cortisol and Organ Transplantation:

Navigating the impact of cortisol on organ transplantation requires a comprehensive approach. Here are some strategies to consider:

Pre-Transplant Evaluation:

Assessing cortisol levels as part of the pre-transplant evaluation can provide valuable information about the patient's stress response and potential risks. Understanding the patient's cortisol status allows healthcare providers to tailor immunosuppressive regimens and develop strategies to manage stress effectively during the transplantation process.

Immunosuppression Management:

The use of corticosteroids and other immunosuppressive medications is an integral part of the post-transplant management. However, minimizing the reliance on corticosteroids whenever possible can help reduce the risk of long-term side effects. Advancements in transplant medicine have led to the development of alternative immunosuppressive strategies that aim to reduce corticosteroid dependence while maintaining adequate immune suppression.

Stress Management and Support:

Psychological support and stress management techniques are crucial for individuals undergoing organ transplantation. Implementing stress-reduction strategies such as mindfulness meditation, relaxation exercises, and counseling can help regulate cortisol levels, promote psychological well-being, and improve overall transplant outcomes. Engaging in support groups and connecting with others who have undergone transplantation can provide valuable emotional support during this challenging journey.

Lifestyle Modifications:

Adopting a healthy lifestyle before and after transplantation can positively impact cortisol levels and overall health. Regular exercise, a balanced diet, adequate sleep, and avoiding smoking and excessive ... consumption can contribute to stress reduction and improved immune function. Consultation with healthcare professionals is important to determine individualized exercise and dietary recommendations based on the specific organ transplantation and overall health status.

So,

Understanding the impact of cortisol on organ transplantation provides valuable insights into the intricate relationship between stress, the immune system, and transplant outcomes. By optimizing cortisol regulation, managing stress, and individualizing immunosuppressive regimens, healthcare providers and patients can work together to enhance transplant success rates and improve the long-term well-being of transplant recipients. Additionally, fostering a supportive environment that addresses the psychological and emotional needs of both recipients and donors is essential for navigating the challenges of organ transplantation.

It's important to note that this chapter provides insights into the potential relationship between cortisol and organ transplantation. However, it should not replace professional medical advice or assessment. Each transplant case is unique, and individualized care is necessary for optimal outcomes. If you have specific concerns or questions related to organ transplantation or the impact of cortisol, consult with your healthcare provider or transplant specialist who can provide personalized guidance based on your specific circumstances.

Chapter 84: The Intricate Dance of Cortisol and Hormonal Changes During the Menstrual Cycle

We will explore the fascinating interplay between cortisol and the body's response to hormonal changes during the menstrual cycle. The menstrual cycle is a complex, beautifully orchestrated process that involves the interplay of various hormones to prepare the body for potential pregnancy. Cortisol, often referred to as the "stress hormone," is intimately connected to the hormonal fluctuations that occur throughout the menstrual cycle. In this chapter, we will delve into the intricate relationship between cortisol and the menstrual cycle, examining how cortisol influences hormonal changes and the impact of stress on menstrual health.

Understanding the Menstrual Cycle:

The menstrual cycle is a natural, cyclical process that occurs in reproductive-age individuals with the goal of preparing the body for potential pregnancy. It typically lasts around 28 days, although cycle length can vary among individuals. The menstrual cycle is regulated by a delicate interplay of hormones, including estrogen, progesterone, follicle-stimulating hormone (FSH), luteinizing hormone (LH), and, yes, cortisol.

Hormonal Changes During the Menstrual Cycle:

The menstrual cycle consists of several distinct phases, each characterized by specific hormonal changes and physiological events. Let's take a closer look at these phases and the hormonal fluctuations that occur:

Menstrual Phase:

The menstrual phase marks the beginning of the cycle and is characterized by the shedding of the uterine lining, resulting in menstrual bleeding. During this phase, hormone levels, including estrogen and progesterone, are relatively low. Cortisol levels may vary, but they generally remain within the normal range during this phase.

Follicular Phase:

The follicular phase follows the menstrual phase and is characterized by the growth and development of ovarian follicles. FSH levels rise, stimulating the maturation of follicles and the production of estrogen. Cortisol levels may fluctuate during this phase, influenced by factors such as stress, lifestyle, and overall health.

Ovulation:

Ovulation marks the release of a mature egg from the ovary. It occurs approximately midway through the menstrual cycle. The surge in LH triggers ovulation, and estrogen levels reach their peak. Cortisol levels may also show some variability during this phase, influenced by factors such as stress and the body's overall stress response.

Luteal Phase:

The luteal phase begins after ovulation and is characterized by the development of the corpus luteum, a temporary endocrine structure that produces progesterone. Progesterone levels rise, preparing the uterus for potential pregnancy. Cortisol levels may fluctuate during this phase, influenced by factors such as stress and the body's stress response.

Cortisol and Hormonal Changes:

Cortisol, as the primary stress hormone, has the potential to influence the delicate hormonal balance during the menstrual cycle. Here are some important considerations:

Stress and Cortisol:

Stress, whether physical, emotional, or environmental, can trigger the release of cortisol as part of the body's stress response. Chronic or prolonged stress can lead to elevated cortisol levels, which may impact the menstrual cycle. High levels of cortisol can disrupt the normal hormonal fluctuations, potentially affecting the timing of ovulation, menstrual regularity, and overall reproductive health.

Cortisol and Hormone Interactions:

Cortisol can interact with other hormones involved in the menstrual cycle, such as estrogen and progesterone. Cortisol can influence the production, metabolism, and clearance of these hormones, potentially altering their levels and affecting the overall hormonal balance. Imbalances in estrogen and progesterone can lead to menstrual irregularities, mood changes, and other menstrual-related symptoms.

Cortisol and Menstrual Symptoms:

Elevated cortisol levels, particularly in the presence of stress, can exacerbate menstrual symptoms such as cramps, bloating, mood swings, and fatigue. Stress-induced cortisol release can amplify the perception of pain and discomfort during menstruation, making symptoms feel more intense.

Navigating Cortisol and the Menstrual Cycle:

Managing cortisol levels and minimizing the impact of stress on the menstrual cycle is crucial for maintaining reproductive health and overall well-being. Here are some strategies to consider:

Stress Management Techniques:

Implement stress management techniques to reduce the impact of stress on cortisol levels and the menstrual cycle. Engage in activities that promote relaxation, such as yoga, meditation, deep breathing exercises, or mindfulness practices. Prioritize self-care, engage in hobbies, and create a supportive social network to help manage stress more effectively.

Regular Exercise:

Regular physical activity has been shown to help reduce stress and promote hormonal balance. Engaging in moderate exercise, such as brisk walking, cycling, or dancing, can have positive effects on cortisol levels and overall menstrual health. Consult with a healthcare professional to determine the exercise regimen that suits your individual needs.

Healthy Lifestyle:

Adopting a healthy lifestyle can positively impact cortisol levels and the menstrual cycle. Ensure you get adequate sleep, eat a balanced diet rich in whole foods, and stay hydrated. Limit caffeine and ... consumption, as they can affect cortisol levels and potentially disrupt hormonal balance.

Seeking Support:

If you experience persistent or severe menstrual irregularities, pain, or other concerns related to the menstrual cycle, seek support from healthcare professionals specializing in reproductive health. They can evaluate your specific situation, provide personalized guidance, and offer appropriate interventions or treatments if necessary.

So,

Understanding the intricate dance between cortisol and hormonal changes during the menstrual cycle provides valuable insights into the impact of stress on reproductive health. By managing stress, promoting self-care, and prioritizing a healthy lifestyle, individuals can help maintain a balanced menstrual cycle and optimize their overall well-being. Remember, everyone's menstrual cycle is unique, and it's essential to listen to your body and seek professional guidance when needed.

Please note that this chapter provides insights into the potential relationship between cortisol and the menstrual cycle. However, it should not replace professional medical advice or assessment. If you have specific concerns or questions related to your menstrual cycle or the impact of cortisol, consult with a healthcare provider or gynecologist who can provide personalized guidance based on your specific circumstances.

Chapter 85: Exploring the Connection Between Cortisol and Crohn's Disease

We will delve into the intriguing relationship between cortisol and the development and progression of Crohn's disease. Crohn's disease is a chronic inflammatory bowel disease that affects the gastrointestinal tract, causing a range of symptoms and complications. Cortisol, known as the "stress hormone," plays a significant role in regulating the body's stress response and immune function. In this chapter, we will explore the complex interactions between cortisol and Crohn's disease, examining its potential impact on disease onset, symptoms, and management strategies.

Understanding Crohn's Disease:

Crohn's disease is a chronic inflammatory condition that primarily affects the gastrointestinal tract, although it can also involve other parts of the body. It is characterized by inflammation that extends deep into the layers of the intestinal walls, leading to various symptoms such as abdominal pain, diarrhea, fatigue, weight loss, and malnutrition. The exact cause of Crohn's disease remains unknown, but it is thought to involve a combination of genetic, environmental, and immune-related factors.

The Role of Cortisol in Crohn's Disease:

Cortisol, as a key hormone involved in the stress response, exerts profound effects on the immune system and inflammation. Here are some important considerations regarding the role of cortisol in Crohn's disease:

Immune Response and Inflammation:

Crohn's disease is characterized by an overactive immune response and chronic inflammation in the gastrointestinal tract. Cortisol, as a potent anti-inflammatory hormone, helps regulate immune function and dampen excessive inflammation. However, in individuals with Crohn's disease, the immune system's response may be dysregulated, leading to imbalances in cortisol production and signaling, potentially exacerbating inflammation.

Cortisol and Stress:

Stress, whether physical, emotional, or psychological, can trigger the release of cortisol as part of the body's stress response. While acute stress may have temporary effects on the immune system, chronic or prolonged stress can disrupt the delicate balance and lead to persistent cortisol dysregulation. In individuals with Crohn's disease, stress-induced cortisol fluctuations may impact disease activity, symptom severity, and overall quality of life.

Cortisol and Intestinal Permeability:

Intestinal permeability, often referred to as "leaky gut," is a common feature of Crohn's disease. It refers to increased permeability of the intestinal lining, allowing substances to pass through more easily. Cortisol can influence intestinal barrier function, and disruptions in cortisol regulation may contribute to increased intestinal permeability in individuals with Crohn's disease, potentially facilitating the entry of harmful substances and triggering immune responses.

Glucocorticoid Therapy:

Glucocorticoids, such as prednisone and hydrocortisone, are synthetic versions of cortisol and are commonly used in the management of Crohn's disease flare-ups. These medications have potent anti-inflammatory properties and can help reduce inflammation and alleviate symptoms. However, long-term use of glucocorticoids can have significant side effects, including weight gain, osteoporosis, diabetes, and immune suppression.

Managing Cortisol and Crohn's Disease:

Managing cortisol levels and minimizing the impact of stress on Crohn's disease is crucial for maintaining disease control and overall well-being. Here are some strategies to consider:

Stress Management Techniques:

Implement stress management techniques to reduce the impact of stress on cortisol levels and disease activity. Engage in activities such as yoga, meditation, deep breathing exercises, or mindfulness practices to help promote relaxation and reduce stress. Counseling or therapy sessions may also be beneficial in developing coping strategies and enhancing emotional well-being.

Lifestyle Modifications:

Adopting a healthy lifestyle can positively impact cortisol levels and Crohn's disease management. Ensure you prioritize adequate sleep, engage in regular physical activity, maintain a balanced diet rich in nutrients, and avoid triggers such as smoking and excessive ... consumption. These lifestyle modifications can help support immune function, reduce inflammation, and improve overall health.

Medication Management:

Work closely with your healthcare provider to develop an individualized treatment plan that minimizes reliance on glucocorticoid medications while effectively managing disease activity. Explore alternative treatment options such as immunomodulators, biologic therapies, and targeted medications that aim to suppress inflammation and promote remission.

Nutritional Support:

Nutrition plays a crucial role in managing Crohn's disease. Work with a registered dietitian or healthcare professional specializing in gastrointestinal disorders to develop a personalized nutrition plan that addresses your specific needs. A balanced diet rich in nutrients can support immune function, reduce inflammation, and promote gut healing.

Support Networks:

Engaging with support networks, such as patient advocacy groups or support groups for individuals with Crohn's disease, can provide valuable emotional support, information, and resources. Connecting with others who share similar experiences can help reduce feelings of isolation and provide a platform for sharing coping strategies and success stories.

So,

Understanding the intricate relationship between cortisol and Crohn's disease sheds light on the potential impact of stress and cortisol dysregulation on disease activity and management. By managing stress, adopting a healthy lifestyle, and working closely with healthcare professionals, individuals with Crohn's disease can strive to optimize their overall well-being and minimize the potential impact of cortisol on disease progression. Remember, each person's experience with Crohn's disease is unique, and it is essential to work with healthcare providers to develop an individualized treatment plan that addresses your specific needs and goals. Through a comprehensive approach that considers both medical interventions and lifestyle modifications, individuals with Crohn's disease can strive for symptom control, improved quality of life, and long-term disease management.

Chapter 86: Unraveling the Impact of Endocrine-Disrupting Chemicals on Cortisol Levels

We will delve into the intriguing connection between exposure to endocrine-disrupting chemicals (EDCs) and cortisol levels. Endocrine-disrupting chemicals are substances found in various products, foods, and environmental pollutants that have the potential to interfere with the normal function of hormones in the body. Cortisol, the primary stress hormone, plays a vital role in regulating many physiological processes. In this chapter, we explore the impact of EDCs on cortisol levels and the potential health implications associated with their exposure.

Understanding Endocrine-Disrupting Chemicals:

Endocrine-disrupting chemicals are substances that mimic, block, or interfere with the body's natural hormones, leading to hormonal imbalances and disruptions in various physiological functions. These chemicals can be found in everyday products such as plastics, pesticides, personal care products, food additives, and industrial pollutants. They have been linked to a range of health concerns, including reproductive disorders, developmental abnormalities, metabolic disturbances, and immune dysfunction.

The Role of Cortisol in the Body:

Cortisol, often referred to as the "stress hormone," is produced by the adrenal glands in response to stress and plays a critical role in the body's stress response and regulation of metabolism, immune function, inflammation, and energy balance. Cortisol levels fluctuate throughout the day, with the highest levels typically in the morning and the lowest at night. Maintaining a delicate balance of cortisol is essential for overall health and well-being.

The Impact of Endocrine-Disrupting Chemicals on Cortisol Levels:

Several studies have suggested that exposure to endocrine-disrupting chemicals may influence cortisol levels. Here are some important considerations:

Disruption of the Hypothalamic-Pituitary-Adrenal (HPA) Axis:

The HPA axis, a complex network involving the hypothalamus, pituitary gland, and adrenal glands, regulates cortisol production and release. Endocrine-disrupting chemicals can disrupt the HPA axis, potentially leading to dysregulation of cortisol levels. Some EDCs have been shown to interfere with the production, metabolism, and clearance of cortisol, contributing to altered cortisol patterns throughout the day.

Stress Response and Cortisol Dysregulation:

Exposure to certain endocrine-disrupting chemicals may trigger stress responses in the body, leading to an increase in cortisol production. Chronic or prolonged exposure to EDCs, particularly those that mimic or block hormonal signals, can disrupt the normal feedback mechanisms that regulate cortisol secretion, leading to chronic cortisol dysregulation and potential health consequences.

Impact on Cortisol Metabolism:

Endocrine-disrupting chemicals can interfere with the enzymes and processes involved in cortisol metabolism. This can result in altered clearance rates of cortisol from the body, leading to prolonged exposure to the hormone and potential imbalances. Altered cortisol metabolism may contribute to a range of health effects, including immune dysfunction, metabolic disturbances, and increased susceptibility to stress-related disorders.

Developmental and Long-Term Effects:

Exposure to endocrine-disrupting chemicals during critical developmental periods, such as pregnancy or early childhood, may have long-lasting effects on cortisol regulation. Disruptions in cortisol levels during sensitive developmental stages can have implications for brain development, immune function, and overall health later in life.

Navigating EDC Exposure and Cortisol Regulation:

While it may be challenging to completely avoid exposure to endocrine-disrupting chemicals in today's world, there are steps you can take to minimize your exposure and support cortisol regulation:

Reduce Exposure to EDCs:

Make informed choices about the products you use and the foods you consume. Opt for organic and locally sourced foods whenever possible to minimize pesticide exposure. Choose personal care products, cleaning agents, and household items that are free from harmful chemicals such as phthalates, parabens, and bisphenol A (BPA). Be mindful of plastic use, especially when it comes to food and beverage containers.

Support Detoxification and Elimination:

A healthy lifestyle that supports the body's detoxification and elimination processes can help reduce the burden of EDCs. Stay hydrated, eat a nutrient-rich diet with plenty of fruits and vegetables, engage in regular physical activity, and consider incorporating practices that promote detoxification, such as sauna sessions or herbal teas that support liver function.

Stress Management:

Since stress can influence cortisol levels and EDCs have the potential to disrupt cortisol regulation, it is crucial to implement stress management techniques. Engage in activities such as meditation, yoga, deep breathing exercises, or mindfulness practices to help reduce stress and support healthy cortisol levels.

Advocate for Policy Changes:

Support efforts aimed at stricter regulations and monitoring of endocrine-disrupting chemicals. Stay informed about emerging research and policy initiatives that focus on reducing EDC exposure in consumer products, agriculture, and industrial practices. By raising awareness and advocating for change, you contribute to a healthier environment for future generations.

So,

The relationship between endocrine-disrupting chemicals and cortisol levels is a complex and evolving field of study. While research has shown potential links between EDC exposure and cortisol dysregulation, further investigation is needed to fully understand the mechanisms and long-term consequences. However, taking steps to minimize exposure to endocrine-disrupting chemicals and support cortisol regulation can contribute to overall health and well-being. By making informed choices, adopting a healthy lifestyle, and advocating for change, we can work towards creating a safer environment for ourselves and future generations. Remember, if you have concerns about EDC exposure or cortisol regulation, consult with healthcare professionals who can provide personalized guidance based on your specific circumstances. Together, we can strive for a healthier and more balanced future.

Chapter 87: Understanding the Connection Between Cortisol and Post-Traumatic Stress Disorder (PTSD)

We will explore the intricate relationship between cortisol and post-traumatic stress disorder (PTSD). PTSD is a complex mental health condition that can develop in individuals who have experienced or witnessed a traumatic event. Cortisol, often referred to as the "stress hormone," plays a significant role in the body's stress response and regulation of emotional and physiological reactions. In this chapter, we delve into the impact of cortisol on the development, symptoms, and treatment of PTSD.

Understanding Post-Traumatic Stress Disorder:

Post-traumatic stress disorder is a psychological condition that can occur following exposure to a traumatic event, such as combat, natural disasters, sexual assault, or accidents. People with PTSD often experience intrusive memories, flashbacks, nightmares, emotional distress, and hypervigilance. The condition can significantly impact their daily functioning, relationships, and overall quality of life. The exact causes of PTSD are complex and can involve genetic, environmental, and biological factors.

The Role of Cortisol in PTSD:

Cortisol plays a vital role in the body's stress response and regulation of emotions and memory. Here are some important considerations regarding the relationship between cortisol and PTSD:

Acute Stress Response:

When a traumatic event occurs, the body's stress response is activated, leading to the release of cortisol. In the immediate aftermath of trauma, cortisol levels are typically elevated, helping the body cope with the stressor. This acute stress response can enhance memory formation, facilitate adaptive responses, and promote recovery.

Cortisol Regulation and Dysregulation:

In individuals with PTSD, cortisol regulation can be disrupted, leading to abnormal cortisol patterns. Studies have shown that some individuals with PTSD may exhibit lower baseline cortisol levels or a blunted cortisol response to stress. Others may experience exaggerated or prolonged cortisol responses. These cortisol dysregulations can contribute to the development and maintenance of PTSD symptoms.

Hippocampal and Amygdala Interplay:

The hippocampus and amygdala, two key brain regions involved in memory and emotion regulation, play a crucial role in the stress response and the development of PTSD. Cortisol interacts with these brain regions, influencing their functioning. Chronic elevation or dysregulation of cortisol can impact the size and functioning of the hippocampus, which is responsible for memory consolidation, and the amygdala, which processes emotional responses. These alterations may contribute to the development and persistence of PTSD symptoms.

Impact on Memory and Emotional Processing:

Cortisol has profound effects on memory and emotional processing. In individuals with PTSD, cortisol dysregulation can affect memory consolidation and retrieval processes, leading to fragmented memories or the formation of intrusive memories and flashbacks. Additionally, cortisol dysregulation may contribute to difficulties in emotional regulation, leading to heightened emotional reactivity and the persistence of negative emotions associated with trauma.

Treatment Implications and Strategies:

Understanding the relationship between cortisol and PTSD can inform treatment approaches and strategies for managing symptoms. Here are some considerations:

Cognitive-Behavioral Therapy (CBT):

CBT is a widely used therapeutic approach for PTSD. It focuses on identifying and challenging negative thought patterns and behaviors associated with trauma. CBT can help individuals develop coping skills, restructure distorted beliefs, and regulate emotional responses. By addressing maladaptive cognitive patterns, CBT may contribute to cortisol regulation and symptom reduction.

Exposure Therapy:

Exposure therapy is another evidence-based treatment for PTSD. It involves gradually exposing individuals to trauma-related stimuli or memories in a safe and controlled environment. This exposure allows individuals to confront their fears and learn new associations with traumatic memories, facilitating the processing and integration of traumatic experiences. Exposure therapy has shown promise in normalizing cortisol responses in individuals with PTSD.

Pharmacological Interventions:

Medications may be prescribed to manage specific symptoms of PTSD, such as anxiety, depression, and sleep disturbances. Some medications, such as selective serotonin reuptake inhibitors (SSRIs), have been shown to regulate cortisol levels and alleviate symptoms. However, medication should be considered in conjunction with therapy and under the guidance of a healthcare professional.

Stress Management Techniques:

Incorporating stress management techniques into daily life can help regulate cortisol levels and support overall well-being. Engage in activities such as mindfulness meditation, deep breathing exercises, yoga, or regular physical exercise to reduce stress and promote relaxation. These practices can positively influence cortisol regulation and contribute to symptom management.

Social Support and Connection:

Social support is crucial in the recovery from PTSD. Maintaining strong relationships with family, friends, and support networks can help reduce feelings of isolation and provide a sense of safety and understanding. Sharing experiences and emotions with trusted individuals can alleviate stress, promote emotional regulation, and contribute to cortisol regulation.

So,

The intricate interplay between cortisol and post-traumatic stress disorder highlights the significant role that stress hormones play in the development and maintenance of PTSD symptoms. Understanding this relationship can inform treatment approaches, strategies for symptom management, and the development of personalized interventions. By incorporating evidence-based therapies, stress management techniques, and social support networks, individuals with PTSD can work towards symptom reduction, improved emotional regulation, and enhanced overall well-being. It is essential to remember that everyone's experience with PTSD is unique, and treatment should be tailored to individual needs and preferences. If you or someone you know is struggling with PTSD, reach out to mental health professionals who can provide guidance, support, and evidence-based interventions. Together, we can foster a greater understanding of the connection between cortisol and PTSD and work towards effective treatments and improved outcomes for individuals affected by this challenging condition.

Chapter 88: Unraveling the Impact of Cortisol on the Body's Response to Chronic Kidney Disease

We will explore the intricate relationship between cortisol and chronic kidney disease (CKD). Chronic kidney disease is a progressive condition that affects the kidneys' ability to function properly over time. Cortisol, often known as the "stress hormone," plays a significant role in various physiological processes and can have both beneficial and detrimental effects on the body. In this chapter, we delve into the impact of cortisol on the development, progression, and management of chronic kidney disease.

Understanding Chronic Kidney Disease:

Chronic kidney disease is a long-term condition characterized by the gradual loss of kidney function. It can result from various factors, including diabetes, high blood pressure, certain medications, autoimmune disorders, and genetic factors. As kidney function declines, waste products and excess fluid accumulate in the body, leading to a range of symptoms and complications, including fatigue, fluid retention, electrolyte imbalances, anemia, and bone disorders.

The Role of Cortisol in Chronic Kidney Disease:

Cortisol, a hormone produced by the adrenal glands, serves several essential functions in the body. Here are some important considerations regarding the relationship between cortisol and chronic kidney disease:

Inflammation and Fibrosis:

Cortisol can have both anti-inflammatory and pro-inflammatory effects on the body. In the context of chronic kidney disease, ongoing inflammation and fibrosis contribute to the progression of kidney damage. Cortisol's anti-inflammatory properties may help reduce inflammation and protect the kidneys from further damage. However, excessive, or prolonged cortisol exposure can promote inflammation and fibrosis, exacerbating kidney injury.

Glucose Metabolism:

Cortisol plays a crucial role in regulating glucose metabolism. In individuals with chronic kidney disease, abnormalities in glucose metabolism are common, including insulin resistance and impaired glucose tolerance. Elevated cortisol levels can contribute to these metabolic disturbances, leading to further complications such as diabetes and cardiovascular disease.

Fluid and Electrolyte Balance:

Maintaining fluid and electrolyte balance is a critical function of the kidneys. Cortisol affects the reabsorption and excretion of sodium and water in the kidneys, thereby influencing fluid balance. In individuals with chronic kidney disease, cortisol dysregulation can disrupt this delicate balance, leading to fluid retention and electrolyte imbalances, such as high blood pressure and edema.

Bone Health:

Cortisol has significant effects on bone health and calcium regulation. In chronic kidney disease, abnormalities in mineral and bone metabolism are prevalent, leading to bone loss and an increased risk of fractures. Elevated cortisol levels can further contribute to bone loss by impairing bone formation and increasing bone resorption, exacerbating the bone-related complications associated with chronic kidney disease.

Management Strategies:

Considering the impact of cortisol on chronic kidney disease, managing cortisol levels and its effects can be beneficial. Here are some strategies:

Blood Pressure Control:

Controlling blood pressure is crucial in managing chronic kidney disease. Elevated cortisol levels can contribute to hypertension, which can further damage the kidneys. Lifestyle modifications, such as a healthy diet low in sodium, regular physical activity, and stress management techniques, can help regulate cortisol levels and support blood pressure control.

Glucose Control:

For individuals with chronic kidney disease and co-existing diabetes or impaired glucose metabolism, managing blood glucose levels is essential. This can be achieved through medication, dietary modifications, regular exercise, and stress reduction techniques. By stabilizing glucose levels, cortisol dysregulation can be minimized, leading to improved overall metabolic control.

Nutritional Support:

A well-balanced diet tailored to the specific nutritional needs of individuals with chronic kidney disease can help minimize cortisol dysregulation and support overall kidney health. Adequate protein intake, appropriate fluid management, and sufficient intake of vitamins and minerals can contribute to hormonal balance and alleviate some of the stress on the kidneys.

Stress Management:

Stress can impact cortisol levels and exacerbate the symptoms of chronic kidney disease. Engaging in stress management techniques, such as relaxation exercises, meditation, yoga, and counseling, can help reduce stress and support cortisol regulation. These practices can positively influence overall well-being and may indirectly benefit kidney health.

Medication Adjustments:

In some cases, medications that impact cortisol levels may need to be adjusted or carefully monitored in individuals with chronic kidney disease. This should be done in consultation with healthcare professionals to ensure the medications are effectively managing cortisol levels while considering their impact on kidney function.
So,
Understanding the intricate relationship between cortisol and chronic kidney disease provides valuable insights into the complex mechanisms underlying this condition. While cortisol dysregulation can contribute to the progression of kidney damage and associated complications, various strategies can be implemented to manage cortisol levels and support overall kidney health. Through lifestyle modifications, stress management techniques, and appropriate medical interventions, individuals with chronic kidney disease can work towards slowing disease progression, managing symptoms, and improving their quality of life. As always, it is important to consult with healthcare professionals who can provide personalized guidance and support throughout the journey of managing chronic kidney disease and cortisol regulation.

Chapter 89: Unveiling the Relationship Between Cortisol and Parkinson's Disease

We will delve into the intriguing connection between cortisol and Parkinson's disease. Parkinson's disease is a progressive neurodegenerative disorder characterized by the loss of dopamine-producing cells in the brain. Cortisol, known as the "stress hormone," is involved in various physiological processes and plays a significant role in the body's stress response. In this chapter, we explore the impact of cortisol on the development, progression, and management of Parkinson's disease.

Understanding Parkinson's Disease:

Parkinson's disease is a complex neurological condition that primarily affects movement and is characterized by symptoms such as tremors, stiffness, bradykinesia (slowed movement), and postural instability. It occurs when dopamine-producing cells in the substantia nigra region of the brain gradually degenerate, leading to a deficiency of dopamine, a neurotransmitter involved in movement control. The exact causes of Parkinson's disease are not fully understood, but a combination of genetic, environmental, and lifestyle factors is thought to contribute to its development.

The Role of Cortisol in Parkinson's Disease:

Cortisol plays a crucial role in various physiological processes, including the regulation of metabolism, immune function, and stress response. Here are some important considerations regarding the relationship between cortisol and Parkinson's disease:

Inflammation and Oxidative Stress:

Inflammation and oxidative stress are believed to play a role in the neurodegenerative processes of Parkinson's disease. Cortisol, as a potent anti-inflammatory and immunosuppressive hormone, can help regulate the body's response to inflammation. However, prolonged, or excessive cortisol release can lead to chronic inflammation and increased oxidative stress, which may contribute to the progression of Parkinson's disease.

Cortisol Dysregulation:

Studies have shown that individuals with Parkinson's disease often exhibit altered cortisol levels and patterns. Some research suggests that individuals with Parkinson's disease may have higher baseline cortisol levels and a blunted cortisol response to stress. Cortisol dysregulation can impact the delicate balance of neurotransmitters, including dopamine, in the brain and potentially contribute to motor and non-motor symptoms of Parkinson's disease.

Stress and Parkinson's Disease:

Stress can have a significant impact on Parkinson's disease. Stressful events, such as major life changes or trauma, may exacerbate symptoms and worsen disease progression. Cortisol, being a key player in the body's stress response, influences the body's physiological and psychological reactions to stressors. Elevated cortisol levels during stressful periods may affect dopaminergic pathways and contribute to symptom fluctuations in individuals with Parkinson's disease.

Impact on Cognitive Function:

Cortisol can also influence cognitive function, which is commonly affected in Parkinson's disease. Excess cortisol levels or chronic cortisol dysregulation may contribute to cognitive impairments, such as difficulties with attention, memory, and executive functioning. The interaction between cortisol and brain regions involved in cognition, such as the hippocampus and prefrontal cortex, may play a role in the cognitive decline associated with Parkinson's disease.

Management Strategies:

Considering the impact of cortisol on Parkinson's disease, managing cortisol levels and its effects can be beneficial. Here are some strategies:

Stress Reduction Techniques:

Engaging in stress reduction techniques can help regulate cortisol levels and alleviate symptoms associated with Parkinson's disease. Techniques such as mindfulness meditation, deep breathing exercises, yoga, and tai chi can promote relaxation, improve emotional well-being, and potentially modulate cortisol dysregulation.

Regular Exercise:

Physical exercise has been shown to have positive effects on Parkinson's disease symptoms and overall well-being. Exercise not only enhances physical function but also helps manage stress and cortisol levels. Engaging in regular aerobic exercise, strength training, and activities that promote flexibility and balance can have a beneficial impact on cortisol regulation and Parkinson's disease management.

Supportive Therapies:

Complementary therapies, such as massage therapy, acupuncture, and music therapy, may provide additional support in managing Parkinson's disease symptoms and reducing stress. These therapies can promote relaxation, improve mood, and potentially influence cortisol levels through their effects on the nervous system and stress response.

Medication Adjustments:

Some medications used to manage Parkinson's disease may have an impact on cortisol levels. It is important to work closely with healthcare professionals to monitor medication effects and make any necessary adjustments to ensure optimal management of both Parkinson's disease symptoms and cortisol regulation.

Healthy Lifestyle:

Adopting a healthy lifestyle that includes a balanced diet, sufficient sleep, and avoidance of excessive ... consumption and smoking can contribute to overall well-being and support cortisol regulation. A diet rich in antioxidants and anti-inflammatory foods may be particularly beneficial in managing Parkinson's disease symptoms and potentially modulating cortisol dysregulation.

So,

Understanding the intricate relationship between cortisol and Parkinson's disease provides valuable insights into the complex mechanisms underlying this neurodegenerative condition. While cortisol dysregulation may contribute to the progression of Parkinson's disease, various strategies can be implemented to manage cortisol levels and support overall well-being. By incorporating stress reduction techniques, regular exercise, supportive therapies, medication adjustments, Anda healthy lifestyle, individuals with Parkinson's disease can work towards optimizing cortisol regulation and potentially improve symptom management. It is important to consult with healthcare professionals who specialize in Parkinson's disease to develop a personalized treatment plan that addresses both the motor and non-motor symptoms of the condition. Through a comprehensive approach that considers cortisol regulation alongside other therapeutic interventions, individuals with Parkinson's disease can strive for better quality of life and potentially slow the progression of the disease. Continued research in this area will further deepen our understanding of the interplay between cortisol and Parkinson's disease, leading to more targeted and effective management strategies in the future.

Chapter 90: Unveiling the Impact of Noise Pollution and Traffic Noise on Cortisol Levels

We will explore the intriguing relationship between cortisol levels and exposure to noise pollution, particularly traffic noise. In our bustling modern world, noise has become an ever-present companion, affecting our daily lives in various ways. Noise pollution, especially from sources like traffic, can have significant impacts on our health and well-being. In this chapter, we delve into the fascinating connection between noise exposure and cortisol levels, shedding light on how noise pollution can influence our body's stress response.

Understanding Noise Pollution and Traffic Noise:

Noise pollution refers to the excessive or disturbing noise that can disrupt the natural balance of sound in our environment. It can originate from various sources, such as transportation, construction, industrial activities, and even recreational activities. Traffic noise, in particular, is a common and pervasive form of noise pollution in urban areas, stemming from vehicles' movement on roadways and highways.

The Impact of Noise on Cortisol Levels:

Cortisol, often referred to as the "stress hormone," is a key player in our body's stress response system. It is produced by the adrenal glands and helps regulate a wide range of physiological processes. Here are some important considerations regarding the relationship between noise pollution, traffic noise, and cortisol levels:

Activation of the Stress Response:

Exposure to noise, including traffic noise, can trigger a physiological stress response in our bodies. The sudden or prolonged exposure to loud and disruptive sounds activates the sympathetic nervous system, leading to the release of stress hormones, including cortisol. This cortisol release prepares our body for the fight-or-flight response, increasing heart rate, blood pressure, and alertness.

Chronic Noise Exposure and Cortisol Dysregulation:

When noise exposure becomes chronic or occurs at high intensities, it can lead to long-term cortisol dysregulation. Prolonged exposure to noise pollution, such as traffic noise, can disrupt the natural cortisol rhythm, resulting in elevated cortisol levels throughout the day. This prolonged cortisol elevation can have detrimental effects on our health, including increased risk of cardiovascular problems, metabolic disorders, and immune system dysfunction.

Sleep Disruption:

Traffic noise can be particularly disruptive to our sleep patterns, as it often occurs during nighttime hours when we should be experiencing restful sleep. Sleep disruption caused by traffic noise can result in altered cortisol levels. Disrupted or poor-quality sleep can lead to elevated cortisol levels at night and decreased cortisol suppression during the day, further contributing to cortisol dysregulation.

Psychological Stress:

In addition to the physiological effects, noise pollution, including traffic noise, can induce psychological stress. Continuous exposure to loud and intrusive sounds can cause annoyance, irritability, and emotional distress. These psychological stressors, in turn, can influence cortisol levels, potentially leading to chronic cortisol elevation and its associated health consequences.

Managing the Effects of Noise Pollution:

While it may be challenging to completely eliminate noise pollution from our lives, there are strategies that can help mitigate its impact on cortisol levels and overall well-being:

Environmental Modifications:

Implementing measures to reduce noise exposure can be beneficial. This may involve using soundproofing materials in buildings, installing noise barriers along roads, and promoting urban planning practices that prioritize noise reduction. Taking steps to create quieter living and working environments can help minimize the negative impact of noise pollution on cortisol levels.

Stress Reduction Techniques:

Engaging in stress reduction techniques can help counteract the effects of noise pollution on cortisol levels. Practices such as mindfulness meditation, deep breathing exercises, and yoga can help promote relaxation, alleviate stress, and potentially modulate cortisol dysregulation. These techniques enable us to cultivate a sense of calm and restore balance in the face of noise-related stressors.

Creating Quiet Spaces:

Seeking out and creating quiet spaces can provide respite from noise pollution. Spending time in natural environments, parks, or dedicated quiet zones allows for a break from the constant auditory stimulation and provides an opportunity for cortisol levels to normalize. These quiet spaces can serve as sanctuaries where individuals can unwind, recharge, and find solace amidst the clamor of urban life.

Healthy Lifestyle Habits:

Adopting a healthy lifestyle that includes regular exercise, a balanced diet, and sufficient sleep can support overall well-being and help mitigate the effects of noise pollution on cortisol levels. Regular physical activity and a nutritious diet can help regulate cortisol levels, improve resilience to stress, and enhance sleep quality. Prioritizing restful sleep can aid in maintaining healthy cortisol rhythms and promote optimal physiological functioning.

So,

The relationship between noise pollution, traffic noise, and cortisol levels highlights the intricate interplay between our environment and our body's stress response system. Prolonged exposure to noise pollution, particularly traffic noise, can disrupt cortisol regulation, contributing to long-term health implications. By implementing environmental modifications, engaging in stress reduction techniques, seeking out quiet spaces, and adopting a healthy lifestyle, individuals can better navigate the challenges posed by noise pollution and mitigate its impact on cortisol levels. Striving for a harmonious balance between our auditory environment and our body's stress response is essential for promoting overall well-being and optimal cortisol regulation in the face of our noisy world.

Chapter 91: Unraveling the Influence of Cortisol on the Body's Response to Organ Rejection after Transplantation

We will delve into the fascinating relationship between cortisol and the body's response to organ rejection after transplantation. Organ transplantation is a life-saving medical procedure that can restore health and improve quality of life for individuals with end-stage organ failure. However, the body's immune system recognizes the transplanted organ as foreign, leading to a potential rejection response. In this chapter, we explore the impact of cortisol, the body's stress hormone, on the delicate balance between organ acceptance and rejection.

Understanding Organ Rejection:

Organ rejection occurs when the recipient's immune system recognizes the transplanted organ as foreign and mounts an immune response to eliminate it. This immune response can be classified into three types: hyperacute rejection, acute rejection, and chronic rejection. Each type involves complex interactions between the recipient's immune system and the transplanted organ.

The Role of Cortisol in the Transplantation Process:

Cortisol, produced by the adrenal glands, plays a crucial role in the body's stress response and immune system regulation. Here are key considerations regarding the impact of cortisol on the body's response to organ rejection:

Immunosuppressive Effects:

Cortisol possesses potent immunosuppressive properties. It helps regulate the immune system's activity, preventing it from mounting an excessive response against foreign substances. In the context of organ transplantation, high cortisol levels during the early post-transplant period may contribute to suppressing the recipient's immune system and reducing the risk of organ rejection.

Cortisol and Immune Cell Function:

Cortisol influences various immune cell populations, including T cells, B cells, and natural killer cells, which are key players in the immune response. Elevated cortisol levels can inhibit the activation and proliferation of immune cells, reducing their ability to recognize and attack the transplanted organ. This modulation of immune cell function by cortisol is an essential factor in maintaining organ acceptance.

Cortisol and Inflammation:

Organ rejection involves an inflammatory response, where pro-inflammatory molecules are released, and immune cells infiltrate the transplanted organ. Cortisol has anti-inflammatory properties that help dampen this immune response and minimize the damage to the transplanted organ. By reducing inflammation, cortisol can potentially mitigate the risk of acute rejection.

Cortisol and Chronic Rejection:

Chronic rejection is a long-term complication that can occur months or years after transplantation. It involves gradual damage to the transplanted organ, leading to its functional decline. Cortisol may play a role in chronic rejection through its influence on fibrosis, the formation of scar tissue. Elevated cortisol levels can contribute to tissue fibrosis, which can impact long-term organ function.

Managing Cortisol Levels and Organ Rejection:

Maintaining an appropriate balance of cortisol levels is crucial in the transplantation process to minimize the risk of rejection and optimize long-term organ function. Here are some strategies that healthcare professionals employ:

Immunosuppressive Medications:

Pharmacological interventions, such as immunosuppressive medications, are routinely prescribed to transplant recipients. These medications help suppress the immune system's activity, reducing the risk of organ rejection. Corticosteroids, which are synthetic forms of cortisol, are often used as part of the immunosuppressive regimen to provide additional suppression of the immune response.

Individualized Corticosteroid Therapy:

The use of corticosteroids, including prednisone or methylprednisolone, in transplant patients varies based on factors such as the type of organ transplant, the recipient's immune response, and the presence of other medical conditions. Corticosteroid therapy may be administered in high doses initially and gradually tapered over time to balance the immunosuppressive effects and potential side effects.

Cortisol Monitoring:

Regular monitoring of cortisol levels can help healthcare professionals assess the recipient's stress response and tailor immunosuppressive therapy accordingly. Frequent monitoring allows for adjustments in medication dosage to maintain the delicate balance between immune suppression and the prevention of infection and other complications.

Stress Reduction and Supportive Care:

Minimizing stress and optimizing overall well-being are vital aspects of post-transplant care. Stress management techniques, such as relaxation exercises, counseling, and support groups, can help reduce cortisol levels and promote emotional well-being. A supportive care team can provide guidance and resources to assist recipients in navigating the emotional challenges associated with transplantation.

So,

The interplay between cortisol and the body's response to organ rejection after transplantation is a multifaceted process. Cortisol's immunosuppressive effects, modulation of immune cell function, regulation of inflammation, and potential role in chronic rejection highlight its significance in maintaining organ acceptance. With careful management of cortisol levels through immunosuppressive medications, individualized therapy, cortisol monitoring, and stress reduction techniques, healthcare professionals strive to minimize the risk of organ rejection and optimize long-term transplant outcomes. Continued research in this area will deepen our understanding of the intricate balance between cortisol and the immune response, leading to more personalized and effective approaches to organ transplantation.

Chapter 92: Unraveling the Impact of Cortisol on the Body's Response to Hormonal Changes during the Aging Process

We will delve into the fascinating relationship between cortisol and the body's response to hormonal changes during the aging process. As we age, our bodies undergo a series of hormonal shifts that can influence various aspects of our health and well-being. Cortisol, the primary stress hormone, plays a vital role in regulating our body's stress response and interacts with other hormones in complex ways. In this chapter, we explore how cortisol impacts the body's response to hormonal changes during aging and shed light on its potential effects on overall health.

Hormonal Changes during the Aging Process:

Aging is a natural and complex process characterized by a gradual decline in various hormonal levels and changes in hormone production and regulation. Some key hormonal changes that occur during aging include:

Decline in Growth Hormone:

As we age, the production of growth hormone, which is responsible for tissue repair, muscle growth, and overall body maintenance, decreases. This decline in growth hormone can affect muscle mass, bone density, and metabolism.

Changes in Sex Hormones:

Both men and women experience changes in sex hormone levels as they age. Menopause marks a significant hormonal shift for women, leading to a decline in estrogen and progesterone levels. In men, testosterone levels gradually decrease with age. These hormonal changes can influence reproductive health, bone density, mood, and cognitive function.

Alterations in Thyroid Hormone Levels:

Thyroid hormone production and regulation can also be affected by the aging process. Thyroid function may decline, leading to changes in metabolism, energy levels, and body temperature regulation.

The Role of Cortisol in Hormonal Changes and Aging:

Cortisol, as the body's primary stress hormone, interacts with various other hormones and plays a significant role in the body's response to hormonal changes during aging. Here are some key considerations:

Stress and Cortisol Regulation:

As we age, the body may become more susceptible to stress due to various factors, such as life changes, health conditions, and caregiving responsibilities. Elevated levels of chronic stress can lead to dysregulation of cortisol production and impact the balance of other hormones in the body. This dysregulation may contribute to age-related health conditions.

Cortisol and Growth Hormone:

Cortisol and growth hormone have a complex relationship. While growth hormone promotes tissue repair and maintenance, cortisol can counteract some of its effects. Elevated cortisol levels, especially in response to chronic stress, can inhibit the production and release of growth hormone, potentially affecting muscle mass, bone density, and overall physical well-being.

Cortisol and Sex Hormones:

Cortisol can influence the production and metabolism of sex hormones, such as estrogen, progesterone, and testosterone. Elevated cortisol levels can disrupt the balance of sex hormones, potentially leading to changes in reproductive health, libido, and mood. In women, cortisol imbalances may exacerbate menopausal symptoms, while in men, cortisol dysregulation can contribute to age-related decline in testosterone levels.

Cortisol and Thyroid Function:

Cortisol and thyroid hormones have intricate interactions. Elevated cortisol levels can interfere with the conversion of inactive thyroid hormone (T4) to its active form (T3), leading to suboptimal thyroid function. Thyroid hormone imbalances can influence metabolism, energy levels, and overall well-being.

Managing Cortisol and Hormonal Changes during Aging:

Although hormonal changes are an inherent part of the aging process, there are strategies to support healthy cortisol levels and promote overall well-being during this stage of life:

Stress Management:

Prioritizing stress management techniques can help regulate cortisol levels and minimize the negative impact of chronic stress on hormonal balance. Engaging in activities such as meditation, yoga, deep breathing exercises, and regular physical activity can promote relaxation, reduce stress, and support overall hormonal health.

Balanced Lifestyle:

Adopting a balanced lifestyle that includes a nutritious diet, regular exercise, and sufficient sleep is essential for maintaining hormonal balance. A diet rich in fruits, vegetables, whole grains, and lean proteins can provide essential nutrients to support hormonal health. Regular exercise helps regulate cortisol levels, enhances mood, and supports overall physical and mental well-being.

Hormone Replacement Therapy:

For individuals experiencing significant hormonal imbalances and related symptoms, hormone replacement therapy (HRT) may be a viable option. HRT involves replacing deficient hormones with synthetic or bio-identical hormones to restore hormonal balance and alleviate symptoms. It is important to discuss the potential risks and benefits of HRT with a healthcare professional.

Regular Health Check-ups:

Regular health check-ups, including hormone level assessments, can provide valuable insights into hormonal changes and help guide appropriate interventions. Collaborating with healthcare professionals who specialize in hormone health and aging can ensure personalized care and support throughout the aging process.

So,

The intricate interplay between cortisol and hormonal changes during the aging process underscores the importance of maintaining a balanced approach to overall well-being. While hormonal changes are natural during aging, chronic stress and cortisol dysregulation can influence the body's response to these changes. By adopting stress management techniques, leading a balanced lifestyle, considering hormone replacement therapy, and staying proactive with regular health check-ups, individuals can support healthy cortisol levels and optimize hormonal balance during the aging process. Understanding the complexities of cortisol's impact on the body's response to hormonal changes empowers individuals to make informed decisions and take proactive steps towards maintaining their health and well-being as they age. By nurturing a holistic approach to health, individuals can embrace the aging process with vitality, resilience, and a sense of empowerment.

Chapter 93: Unraveling the Role of Cortisol in the Development and Progression of Ulcerative Colitis

We will delve into the intriguing relationship between cortisol and the development and progression of ulcerative colitis. Ulcerative colitis is a chronic inflammatory bowel disease that affects the colon and rectum, causing symptoms such as abdominal pain, diarrhea, and rectal bleeding. While the exact cause of ulcerative colitis is still unknown, research suggests that various factors, including genetics, immune system dysfunction, and environmental triggers, contribute to its development. In this chapter, we explore the role of cortisol, the primary stress hormone, in the pathogenesis and progression of ulcerative colitis, shedding light on its potential impact on the disease.

Understanding Ulcerative Colitis:

Before we delve into the role of cortisol, let's gain a basic understanding of ulcerative colitis. Ulcerative colitis is characterized by chronic inflammation of the inner lining of the colon and rectum. This inflammation typically starts in the rectum and spreads to other parts of the colon. The exact cause of ulcerative colitis remains elusive, but it is believed to result from an abnormal immune response in genetically susceptible individuals triggered by environmental factors, such as diet and stress.

The Role of Cortisol in the Immune Response:

Cortisol, commonly known as the stress hormone, is produced by the adrenal glands in response to stress. It plays a crucial role in regulating the immune system and modulating the body's inflammatory response. Cortisol acts as a potent anti-inflammatory agent, dampening the immune system's activity to prevent excessive inflammation. However, under certain circumstances, cortisol dysregulation can occur, leading to an imbalance in the immune response.

Cortisol and Ulcerative Colitis:

Research suggests that cortisol may play a role in the development and progression of ulcerative colitis. Here are some key considerations:

Inflammation and Cortisol:

In ulcerative colitis, the immune system mistakenly triggers an inflammatory response in the colon and rectum, leading to chronic inflammation. Cortisol helps regulate the intensity and duration of the inflammatory response. However, in individuals with ulcerative colitis, cortisol levels may be dysregulated, leading to inadequate control of inflammation, and contributing to the chronicity of the disease.

Cortisol and Stress:

Stress is known to be a triggering factor for ulcerative colitis flare-ups. During periods of stress, cortisol levels rise as part of the body's natural stress response. However, chronic stress can lead to dysregulation of cortisol production, potentially contributing to ongoing inflammation and worsening of ulcerative colitis symptoms.

Cortisol and Gut Barrier Function:

The gut barrier plays a critical role in maintaining the integrity of the intestinal lining and preventing the entry of harmful substances into the bloodstream. Cortisol influences the function of the gut barrier by regulating tight junction proteins and mucus production. Dysregulation of cortisol levels can disrupt the gut barrier, potentially allowing bacteria and other substances to penetrate the intestinal lining and trigger inflammation.

Cortisol and Immune System Dysfunction:

Cortisol plays a complex role in modulating the immune system's response. In individuals with ulcerative colitis, immune system dysfunction is evident, with an exaggerated inflammatory response in the colon. Cortisol dysregulation can further contribute to immune system dysfunction, leading to a cycle of chronic inflammation and tissue damage.

Managing Cortisol and Ulcerative Colitis:

While cortisol dysregulation may be a contributing factor in ulcerative colitis, it's important to note that the disease is multi-faceted, involving various genetic, environmental, and immune-related factors. However, there are strategies to manage cortisol levels and potentially support the management of ulcerative colitis:

Stress Management:

Effective stress management techniques can help regulate cortisol levels and minimize its impact on ulcerative colitis. Engaging in activities such as meditation, deep breathing exercises, yoga, and regular physical exercise can reduce stress levels, promote relaxation, and potentially alleviate symptoms.

Supportive Therapies:

Complementary therapies, such as acupuncture, massage, and cognitive-behavioral therapy, may help individuals manage stress, reduce inflammation, and support overall well-being. These therapies can be used alongside conventional medical treatments to enhance symptom management and improve quality of life.

Medication and Treatment:

Various medications, including anti-inflammatory drugs, immunosuppressants, and biologic therapies, are commonly prescribed to manage ulcerative colitis symptoms and reduce inflammation. Working closely with healthcare professionals can help determine the most appropriate treatment plan, including medications that may help regulate cortisol levels and control disease activity.

Lifestyle Modifications:

Adopting a healthy lifestyle is crucial for individuals with ulcerative colitis. A well-balanced diet that focuses on whole, nutrient-dense foods can provide essential nutrients and support overall gut health. Regular exercise, sufficient sleep, and maintaining a healthy weight can also contribute to overall well-being and potentially help manage cortisol levels.

So,

While the precise role of cortisol in the development and progression of ulcerative colitis is still being elucidated, research suggests that cortisol dysregulation may contribute to immune system dysfunction and chronic inflammation. Managing stress, supporting a healthy lifestyle, and working closely with healthcare professionals are important steps in managing cortisol levels and potentially mitigating the impact of cortisol dysregulation on ulcerative colitis. By taking a holistic approach to ulcerative colitis management, individuals can strive for better symptom control, improved quality of life, and a sense of empowerment in their journey with the disease.

Chapter 94: Unveiling the Impact of Household Chemicals and Cleaning Products on Cortisol Levels

We will explore the intriguing question of whether exposure to household chemicals and cleaning products can influence cortisol levels. In our daily lives, we come into contact with a variety of cleaning agents, detergents, and other household products that contain chemicals. These products are designed to keep our homes clean and hygienic, but could they potentially have an impact on our stress hormone cortisol? In this chapter, we will delve into the potential effects of household chemicals on cortisol levels, shedding light on the importance of understanding the potential risks associated with these everyday products.

Understanding Cortisol:

Before we delve into the relationship between household chemicals and cortisol levels, let's start by understanding cortisol and its role in the body. Cortisol, often referred to as the stress hormone, is produced by the adrenal glands in response to stress. It plays a crucial role in regulating various physiological functions, including metabolism, immune response, and inflammation. Cortisol levels naturally fluctuate throughout the day, with higher levels in the morning and lower levels in the evening.

Household Chemicals and Cortisol:

While research on the specific effects of household chemicals on cortisol levels is limited, several studies have explored the potential impact of environmental chemicals on endocrine function, including cortisol regulation. Here are some key considerations:

Endocrine Disrupting Chemicals (EDCs):

Certain household chemicals and cleaning products contain ingredients that may have endocrine-disrupting properties. These chemicals, known as EDCs, can interfere with the body's hormonal balance and disrupt the normal function of various endocrine glands, including the adrenal glands responsible for cortisol production.

Inhalation and Absorption:

Exposure to household chemicals can occur through inhalation of fumes or absorption through the skin. Some cleaning products release volatile organic compounds (VOCs) into the air, which can be inhaled. These VOCs have been linked to various health concerns, including potential effects on endocrine function. Additionally, when we handle cleaning products, the chemicals can come into contact with our skin, potentially leading to absorption into the bloodstream.

Potential Mechanisms:

The specific mechanisms through which household chemicals may impact cortisol levels are not yet fully understood. However, it is believed that certain chemicals may mimic or interfere with the body's natural hormone signaling pathways, leading to dysregulation of cortisol production and regulation.

Individual Sensitivity:

It is important to note that individuals may vary in their sensitivity to household chemicals. Some people may be more susceptible to the potential effects of these chemicals on cortisol levels, while others may be less affected. Factors such as age, pre-existing health conditions, and genetic variations can influence individual responses to chemical exposure.

Minimizing Exposure and Promoting Well-being:

Given the potential risks associated with household chemicals and their impact on cortisol levels, it is important to adopt practices that minimize exposure and promote overall well-being:

Choose Safer Alternatives:

Consider using environmentally friendly and non-toxic cleaning products. Look for products that are labeled as "green," "eco-friendly," or "naturally derived." These products are typically formulated with fewer harmful chemicals, reducing the potential risk of endocrine disruption.

Ventilation:

Ensure proper ventilation when using cleaning products to minimize inhalation of fumes. Open windows or use exhaust fans to allow fresh air circulation, especially in confined spaces.

Protective Measures:

When handling cleaning products, consider using protective gloves and clothing to minimize direct skin contact. This can help reduce absorption of chemicals into the bloodstream.

Read Labels and Follow Instructions:

Read product labels carefully and follow instructions for use and disposal. This will help you understand the potential risks associated with the chemicals in the product and how to handle them safely.

Establish Cleaning Routines:

Maintain a regular cleaning routine to prevent the buildup of dirt and grime, reducing the need for harsh cleaning products. Simple cleaning practices, such as regular dusting and wiping surfaces with natural cleaners like vinegar or baking soda, can often suffice for day-to-day cleaning.

Prioritize Natural Cleaning Solutions:

Explore natural alternatives for cleaning, such as homemade cleaners using ingredients like lemon juice, vinegar, and baking soda. These options are generally safer and can be effective for many cleaning tasks.

So,

While the specific impact of household chemicals on cortisol levels requires further research, there is growing evidence suggesting a potential link between exposure to certain chemicals and endocrine disruption. Taking steps to minimize exposure to household chemicals and opting for safer alternatives can contribute to a healthier home environment and potentially reduce the risks associated with cortisol dysregulation. By making informed choices and adopting mindful cleaning practices, individuals can create a safer and more harmonious living space while supporting their overall well-being.

Chapter 95: Unveiling the Link Between Cortisol and the Body's Response to Obsessive-Compulsive Disorder (OCD)

We will dive into the intriguing relationship between cortisol and the body's response to obsessive-compulsive disorder (OCD). OCD is a complex mental health condition characterized by intrusive thoughts, obsessions, and repetitive behaviors. While the exact causes of OCD are not fully understood, emerging research suggests that cortisol, a hormone produced by the body in response to stress, may play a role in the development and progression of OCD symptoms. In this chapter, we will explore the interplay between cortisol and OCD, shedding light on the potential mechanisms and implications for understanding and managing this challenging disorder.

Understanding OCD:

Before we delve into the relationship between cortisol and OCD, let's first establish a foundation of understanding about this mental health condition. OCD is a chronic psychiatric disorder that affects people of all ages and can significantly impact their daily lives. Individuals with OCD often experience intrusive thoughts or obsessions that cause anxiety, and they engage in repetitive behaviors or rituals as a way to alleviate distress or prevent feared outcomes. OCD can manifest in various forms, such as compulsive cleaning, excessive checking, or mental rituals.

Cortisol and Stress Response:

Cortisol, often referred to as the stress hormone, is produced by the adrenal glands in response to stress. It plays a vital role in the body's stress response system, helping to regulate energy metabolism, immune function, and inflammation. Cortisol levels naturally fluctuate throughout the day, with higher levels in the morning and lower levels in the evening. However, chronic stress and dysregulation of the stress response system can lead to abnormal cortisol levels, potentially contributing to the development and maintenance of various mental health conditions, including OCD.

The HPA Axis and Cortisol Dysregulation:
The hypothalamic-pituitary-adrenal (HPA) axis is a complex system that regulates the body's stress response, with cortisol being one of the primary hormones involved. In individuals with OCD, there may be alterations in the functioning of the HPA axis, resulting in dysregulated cortisol levels. Several factors contribute to this dysregulation, including genetic predisposition, environmental stressors, and childhood experiences. Research suggests that the dysregulation of cortisol and the HPA axis may contribute to the development and persistence of OCD symptoms.
Cortisol and OCD Symptoms:
While the exact mechanisms underlying the relationship between cortisol and OCD are not fully understood, several hypotheses have been proposed:
Stress and Cortisol Exacerbation:
Stress is known to exacerbate OCD symptoms, and cortisol levels tend to increase during times of stress. Higher cortisol levels may amplify the anxiety and distress associated with OCD, making it more challenging to manage symptoms effectively.
Feedback Loop and Cortisol Resistance:
In some individuals with OCD, there may be a dysregulation in the feedback loop between cortisol and the HPA axis. This dysregulation can lead to reduced sensitivity to cortisol, resulting in an inadequate stress response. This resistance to cortisol may contribute to the persistence of OCD symptoms.
Inflammation and Neurotransmitter Imbalance:
Elevated cortisol levels can also influence the immune system and contribute to inflammation. Inflammation, in turn, has been associated with various mental health disorders, including OCD. Imbalances in neurotransmitters, such as serotonin, dopamine, and glutamate, which are implicated in OCD, may also be influenced by cortisol dysregulation.
Implications for Treatment and Management:
Understanding the relationship between cortisol and OCD can have implications for treatment and management strategies:
Cognitive-Behavioral Therapy (CBT):

CBT, particularly exposure and response prevention (ERP), is a highly effective treatment for OCD. CBT helps individuals confront their fears and gradually reduce their compulsive behaviors. By addressing the underlying anxiety and stress associated with OCD, cortisol dysregulation may be indirectly targeted.

Medication and Cortisol Regulation:

Certain medications, such as selective serotonin reuptake inhibitors (SSRIs), are commonly prescribed to manage OCD symptoms. These medications may indirectly influence cortisol levels by modulating neurotransmitter activity and reducing anxiety.

Stress Management Techniques:

Incorporating stress management techniques into daily life can be beneficial for individuals with OCD. Techniques such as mindfulness, relaxation exercises, regular exercise, and adequate sleep can help regulate cortisol levels and reduce overall stress.

Lifestyle Factors:

Maintaining a healthy lifestyle, including a balanced diet, regular physical activity, and sufficient sleep, can contribute to overall well-being and potentially help regulate cortisol levels.

So,

While the relationship between cortisol and OCD is still being explored, evidence suggests a complex interplay between stress, cortisol dysregulation, and the development and progression of OCD symptoms. By understanding the potential role of cortisol in OCD, we gain valuable insights into the underlying mechanisms and treatment approaches. Further research is needed to elucidate the intricate details of this relationship and develop targeted interventions that address cortisol dysregulation in the context of OCD. By adopting a comprehensive approach that combines psychological interventions, medication, stress management techniques, and healthy lifestyle choices, individuals with OCD can work towards managing their symptoms and improving their overall well-being.

Chapter 96: Unveiling the Impact of Cortisol on the Body's Response to Chronic Obstructive Pulmonary Disease (COPD)

We will explore the fascinating connection between cortisol and the body's response to chronic obstructive pulmonary disease (COPD). COPD is a progressive lung disease characterized by breathing difficulties, coughing, and wheezing. It is primarily caused by long-term exposure to irritants, such as cigarette smoke or environmental pollutants. While the primary mechanisms of COPD involve inflammation and airway obstruction, emerging research suggests that cortisol, the stress hormone, may also play a role in modulating the body's response to COPD. In this chapter, we delve into the intricate relationship between cortisol and COPD, uncovering the potential implications for understanding and managing this chronic respiratory condition.

Understanding COPD:

Before we dive into the connection between cortisol and COPD, let's establish a foundational understanding of this complex respiratory disease. COPD encompasses two main conditions: chronic bronchitis and emphysema. Chronic bronchitis is characterized by inflammation and excess mucus production in the airways, while emphysema involves the destruction of the lung tissue, leading to loss of elasticity and air trapping. COPD is primarily caused by exposure to noxious particles or gases, most commonly from cigarette smoking, but also from occupational or environmental factors.

Cortisol and the Stress Response:

Cortisol, often referred to as the stress hormone, is produced by the adrenal glands in response to stress. It plays a crucial role in regulating the body's stress response, influencing metabolism, inflammation, and immune function. In individuals with COPD, the chronic inflammation and ongoing stress related to the disease may contribute to cortisol dysregulation. Elevated cortisol levels have been observed in some individuals with COPD, potentially affecting various aspects of the disease, including symptom severity, lung function, and overall health outcomes.

Cortisol and COPD Symptoms:

The impact of cortisol on COPD symptoms is multifaceted, involving several mechanisms:

Inflammation and Airway Hyperresponsiveness:

COPD is characterized by chronic inflammation in the airways and lung tissue. Cortisol, as a potent anti-inflammatory hormone, plays a role in modulating this inflammatory response. However, in individuals with COPD, the chronic exposure to inflammation and oxidative stress can lead to cortisol resistance, reducing its effectiveness in controlling inflammation. This may contribute to persistent airway inflammation and hyperresponsiveness, exacerbating COPD symptoms.

Muscle Wasting and Weakness:

COPD is associated with skeletal muscle wasting and weakness, a condition known as muscle cachexia. Cortisol has catabolic effects on muscle tissue, meaning it can contribute to muscle breakdown. Elevated cortisol levels in COPD may exacerbate muscle wasting, leading to further weakness and decreased exercise capacity.

Bone Health and Osteoporosis:

Cortisol also plays a role in bone metabolism. Prolonged exposure to high cortisol levels can lead to bone loss and an increased risk of osteoporosis. In COPD, where individuals may experience reduced physical activity, systemic inflammation, and hormonal imbalances, cortisol dysregulation may further contribute to bone mineral density loss and skeletal complications.

Psychological Impact and Stress:

Living with COPD can be challenging and stressful, both physically and emotionally. The psychological impact of COPD, including anxiety, depression, and reduced quality of life, can affect cortisol regulation. Stressful situations and psychological distress can lead to cortisol dysregulation, potentially exacerbating COPD symptoms and impacting overall well-being.

Implications for Treatment and Management:

Understanding the relationship between cortisol and COPD has implications for treatment and management strategies:

Medications:

Inhaled corticosteroids, a type of medication commonly used in COPD management, aim to reduce airway inflammation. These medications help to counteract the inflammatory processes associated with COPD and may indirectly influence cortisol levels by modulating local inflammation.

Stress Management Techniques:

Incorporating stress management techniques into the daily routine can help individuals with COPD manage cortisol levels and improve overall well-being. Techniques such as relaxation exercises, deep breathing, mindfulness, and engaging in pleasurable activities can help reduce stress and support better cortisol regulation.

Pulmonary Rehabilitation:

Pulmonary rehabilitation programs, a comprehensive approach to COPD management, include exercise training, education, and psychosocial support. These programs can help individuals improve exercise capacity, reduce symptoms, and better cope with the psychological impact of COPD, potentially influencing cortisol regulation.

Lifestyle Factors:

Maintaining a healthy lifestyle is crucial for individuals with COPD. Regular physical activity, a balanced diet, and adequate sleep contribute to overall well-being and may help support optimal cortisol regulation.

So,

While the relationship between cortisol and COPD is a complex interplay of inflammatory processes, hormonal regulation, and stress response, emerging research suggests that cortisol dysregulation may influence various aspects of COPD. Understanding the potential impact of cortisol on COPD symptoms, muscle wasting, bone health, and psychological well-being can inform treatment and management strategies. By adopting a holistic approach that combines medication, stress management techniques, pulmonary rehabilitation, and a healthy lifestyle, individuals with COPD can work towards optimizing their health outcomes and achieving a better quality of life. Ongoing research in this field holds promise for further unraveling the intricate connections between cortisol and COPD, paving the way for more personalized and effective approaches to COPD management in the future.

Chapter 97: The Intriguing Connection Between Cortisol and Amyotrophic Lateral Sclerosis (ALS)

We will embark on a journey to explore the fascinating relationship between cortisol and amyotrophic lateral sclerosis (ALS), a progressive neurodegenerative disease that affects nerve cells in the brain and spinal cord. ALS, also known as Lou Gehrig's disease, leads to the gradual loss of muscle control, impacting speech, movement, and eventually, the ability to breathe. While the exact cause of ALS remains unknown, there is growing interest in understanding the role of cortisol, the stress hormone, in the development and progression of this devastating condition. In this chapter, we delve into the complex interactions between cortisol and ALS, shedding light on their potential implications for understanding and managing this enigmatic disease.

Understanding ALS:

Before we explore the connection between cortisol and ALS, let's establish a foundational understanding of this perplexing neurological disorder. ALS involves the degeneration and death of motor neurons, the nerve cells responsible for controlling voluntary muscle movement. As the motor neurons deteriorate, the muscles they innervate gradually weaken and waste away, leading to progressive loss of muscle function. The causes of ALS are still not fully understood, but a combination of genetic and environmental factors, as well as abnormalities in protein processing and inflammation, are believed to contribute to its development.

Cortisol and the Stress Response:

Cortisol, often referred to as the stress hormone, is produced by the adrenal glands in response to stress. It plays a vital role in regulating the body's stress response, influencing metabolism, immune function, and inflammation. While cortisol is essential for maintaining normal bodily functions, chronically elevated levels or dysregulation of cortisol can have detrimental effects on various body systems.

Cortisol and ALS:

The potential role of cortisol in ALS is a subject of ongoing research and investigation. Here are some of the key aspects being explored:

Neuroinflammation and Oxidative Stress:

Inflammation and oxidative stress are believed to contribute to the degeneration of motor neurons in ALS. Cortisol, with its anti-inflammatory properties, plays a role in modulating the immune response and reducing inflammation. However, in ALS, the chronic inflammation and oxidative stress associated with the disease may lead to dysregulation of cortisol, potentially compromising its anti-inflammatory effects and exacerbating neuroinflammation.

Glutamate Excitotoxicity:

Glutamate, a neurotransmitter, plays a crucial role in transmitting signals between nerve cells. In ALS, there is an imbalance in glutamate levels, leading to excessive stimulation of motor neurons and subsequent cell damage (excitotoxicity). Cortisol may influence glutamate signaling and metabolism, potentially impacting the excitotoxic processes involved in ALS pathogenesis.

Muscle Wasting and Weakness:

ALS is characterized by progressive muscle wasting and weakness. Cortisol has catabolic effects on muscle tissue, meaning it can contribute to muscle breakdown. Elevated cortisol levels in individuals with ALS may further exacerbate muscle wasting and weakness, potentially accelerating the decline in motor function.

Psychological Impact and Stress:

Living with ALS can be emotionally challenging, not only for individuals but also for their families and caregivers. The psychological impact of ALS, including anxiety, depression, and reduced quality of life, can influence cortisol regulation. Stressful situations and psychological distress can lead to cortisol dysregulation, potentially exacerbating ALS symptoms and impacting overall well-being.

Implications for Treatment and Management:

While the precise role of cortisol in ALS is still being elucidated, understanding its potential impact has implications for treatment and management strategies:

Stress Management and Psychological Support:

Given the potential connection between psychological distress and cortisol dysregulation, providing comprehensive psychological support and stress management techniques to individuals with ALS can play a vital role in optimizing their well-being. Techniques such as counseling, mindfulness, relaxation exercises, and support groups can help reduce stress and improve coping mechanisms.

Anti-Inflammatory Approaches:

As neuroinflammation is implicated in ALS, anti-inflammatory strategies may hold promise. Some research suggests that medications targeting inflammation and immune dysregulation may have potential benefits in ALS. By modulating the inflammatory response, these interventions may indirectly influence cortisol regulation.

Nutritional Support:

Maintaining optimal nutrition is essential for individuals with ALS. A balanced diet, rich in nutrients and antioxidants, can support overall health and potentially mitigate the impact of cortisol on muscle wasting. Consultation with a registered dietitian can provide personalized dietary recommendations.

Medications:

Although there is currently no cure for ALS, medications approved for managing symptoms, such as riluzole and edaravone, may indirectly influence cortisol regulation through their effects on disease progression and neuroprotection. Ongoing research aims to identify novel therapeutic targets that may directly or indirectly impact cortisol dysregulation in ALS.

So,

While the precise role of cortisol in the development and progression of ALS is still a topic of investigation, emerging research suggests its potential involvement in neuroinflammation, muscle wasting, and the stress response associated with the disease. Understanding the complex interplay between cortisol and ALS holds promise for shedding light on the underlying mechanisms of this debilitating condition and may pave the way for the development of novel therapeutic approaches. By combining conventional medical management with comprehensive psychological support, stress management techniques, and other interventions that optimize overall well-being, individuals with ALS can navigate the challenges of the disease with enhanced quality of life and potentially improved outcomes. Continued research into the cortisol-ALS relationship will further advance our understanding and help shape future strategies for tackling this devastating neurodegenerative disorder.

Chapter 98: Unveiling the Impact of Indoor Air Pollutants and Mold on Cortisol Levels

We will explore the intriguing connection between indoor air pollutants, mold, and cortisol levels. Indoor environments are not immune to air pollution, and exposure to pollutants and mold can have significant implications for our health. In this chapter, we delve into the effects of indoor air pollutants and mold on cortisol, the stress hormone, and how these interactions may impact our well-being. Understanding the relationship between indoor air quality and cortisol can empower us to make informed decisions about our living spaces and take necessary steps to create healthier environments.

Indoor Air Pollutants: An Unseen Challenge:

Our homes and workplaces should be sanctuaries of safety and comfort, but they can also be reservoirs of hidden pollutants. Indoor air pollutants can originate from various sources, including building materials, cleaning products, furnishings, and even outdoor air contaminants that infiltrate our living spaces. These pollutants can include volatile organic compounds (VOCs), formaldehyde, particulate matter, tobacco smoke, allergens, and chemical residues. Prolonged exposure to these pollutants can have adverse effects on our health, triggering respiratory problems, allergies, asthma, and other respiratory conditions.

Mold: A Silent Intruder:

Another concern in indoor environments is the presence of mold. Mold thrives in damp, poorly ventilated areas, such as basements, bathrooms, and areas affected by water leaks or flooding. It releases spores into the air, which, when inhaled, can cause a range of health issues, including allergic reactions, respiratory symptoms, and even exacerbation of asthma. Mold can also produce mycotoxins, which are toxic compounds that can have detrimental effects on our health.

Cortisol and the Stress Response:

To understand the impact of indoor air pollutants and mold on cortisol levels, we must first grasp the role of cortisol in the stress response. Cortisol is a hormone released by the adrenal glands in response to stress. It helps regulate various physiological processes, including metabolism, immune function, inflammation, and the body's response to threats. Cortisol levels typically follow a diurnal pattern, peaking in the morning and gradually declining throughout the day.

Indoor Air Quality and Cortisol Levels:

Exposure to indoor air pollutants and mold can disrupt the delicate balance of cortisol in several ways:

Inflammation and Immune Response:

Indoor air pollutants, such as VOCs and particulate matter, can trigger an inflammatory response in the body. Inflammation, in turn, can influence cortisol levels, leading to dysregulation. Mold spores and mycotoxins, known for their potential to induce inflammation, can also impact cortisol production and regulation.

Allergic Reactions and Asthma:

Indoor allergens, including mold spores, can provoke allergic reactions and worsen asthma symptoms. Allergies and asthma are associated with increased stress and cortisol levels. The constant activation of the body's immune response and the resulting stress can disrupt cortisol rhythms and contribute to chronic elevation of cortisol levels.

Psychological Stress:

Living in environments contaminated with indoor air pollutants and mold can create psychological stress. Concerns about health risks, odors, and the impact on overall well-being can trigger anxiety and stress responses. Chronic psychological stress can affect cortisol levels, leading to dysregulation and potentially elevated cortisol throughout the day.

Sleep Disruption:

Poor indoor air quality, often accompanied by mold growth, can negatively impact sleep quality. Disrupted sleep patterns and insufficient sleep can disrupt cortisol rhythms and lead to dysregulated cortisol levels.

Managing Indoor Air Quality for Healthy Cortisol Levels:

To promote healthy cortisol levels and create a healthier indoor environment, consider the following measures:

Improve Ventilation:

Ensure proper ventilation in your living spaces. Open windows whenever possible to allow fresh air circulation. Use exhaust fans in kitchens, bathrooms, and other areas prone to moisture and pollutants.

Prevent Moisture and Mold:

Address any moisture issues promptly. Repair leaks, dry wet areas, and reduce humidity levels through dehumidifiers or proper ventilation. Regularly inspect and clean areas prone to mold growth, such as bathrooms, basements, and crawl spaces.

Choose Low-toxicity Products:

Opt for low-toxicity cleaning products, paints, and furnishings. Look for products labeled as low VOC or VOC-free. Be cautious when introducing new furniture or materials into your living spaces and ensure proper off-gassing.

Maintain Cleanliness:

Regularly clean your living spaces, including floors, carpets, and upholstery, to minimize the buildup of dust, allergens, and potential pollutants. Vacuum with a HEPA filter and use damp cleaning methods to capture and remove particles effectively.

Test and Remediate:

If you suspect mold growth, consider testing your indoor air or consulting professionals for mold assessment. If mold is detected, proper remediation measures should be taken to ensure a safe and healthy environment.

Seek Professional Help:

If you or your loved ones experience persistent health symptoms related to indoor air quality, consult with healthcare professionals or environmental specialists who can assess your situation and provide guidance tailored to your needs.

So,

Indoor air pollutants and mold can have a significant impact on our health and well-being, including the regulation of cortisol levels. Understanding the interplay between indoor air quality, cortisol, and our body's stress response empowers us to take proactive steps to create healthier living environments. By improving ventilation, preventing mold growth, choosing low-toxicity products, maintaining cleanliness, and seeking professional assistance when needed, we can reduce exposure to indoor pollutants and mold, promoting healthier cortisol levels and overall well-being. Prioritizing a clean and healthy indoor environment not only benefits our physical health but also contributes to a sense of peace, comfort, and serenity in our daily lives.

Chapter 99: Unraveling the Impact of Cortisol on the Body's Response to Organ Failure and Transplantation

We will delve into the intricate relationship between cortisol and the body's response to organ failure and transplantation. Organ failure can be a life-altering condition, and transplantation offers a ray of hope for those in need. In this chapter, we explore how cortisol, the stress hormone, influences the body's response to organ failure, the transplantation process, and the subsequent journey of the transplanted organ. Understanding the role of cortisol in this context can provide valuable insights into optimizing patient outcomes and improving the success of organ transplantation.

The Significance of Organ Failure:

Organ failure occurs when an organ's ability to function optimally is compromised, leading to a decline in overall health. Common causes of organ failure include chronic diseases, genetic disorders, infections, injuries, and autoimmune conditions. When organ failure becomes irreversible or life-threatening, transplantation may be considered as a treatment option.

The Cortisol-Stress Connection:

To grasp the impact of cortisol on organ failure and transplantation, we must first comprehend the stress response. Cortisol, produced by the adrenal glands, plays a vital role in regulating the body's response to stress. In times of acute or chronic stress, cortisol levels rise to help the body mobilize energy, enhance alertness, and modulate the immune system. However, prolonged, or excessive cortisol release can have detrimental effects on various body systems, including those involved in organ function and transplantation.

Cortisol and Organ Failure:

Immune System Dysfunction:

Elevated cortisol levels associated with chronic stress can impair immune system function. This can lead to increased susceptibility to infections, delayed wound healing, and a higher risk of complications in individuals with organ failure. Moreover, the immune system's response to the transplanted organ can be influenced by cortisol, affecting the success of transplantation.

Metabolic Imbalances:

Cortisol plays a role in regulating glucose metabolism, and chronic elevation of cortisol levels can lead to insulin resistance and impaired glucose control. This can be particularly problematic for individuals with organ failure who may already have underlying metabolic disturbances. Proper management of cortisol levels becomes crucial to mitigate the risk of metabolic imbalances.

Cardiovascular System:

Prolonged cortisol elevation can have adverse effects on the cardiovascular system. It can contribute to hypertension, dyslipidemia, and endothelial dysfunction, all of which can further exacerbate the complications associated with organ failure. Effective cortisol management becomes essential in preserving cardiovascular health in patients with organ failure.

Cortisol and the Transplantation Process:

Pre-transplantation Phase:

Organ transplantation is a complex and demanding process, requiring meticulous evaluation, preparation, and matching of the donor and recipient. During this phase, cortisol levels can be influenced by the anticipation, anxiety, and stress associated with the transplantation journey. High cortisol levels can have implications for patient well-being, immune function, and the body's ability to withstand the surgical procedure.

Perioperative Period:

The surgical procedure itself triggers a significant stress response in the body, leading to a surge in cortisol levels. While this response is a natural part of the body's adaptation to stress, excessive cortisol release can have adverse effects on wound healing, infection risk, and overall recovery. Appropriate perioperative cortisol management is crucial to optimize patient outcomes.

Post-transplantation Phase:

Following transplantation, cortisol levels continue to play a role in the body's response to the newly transplanted organ. Immune system regulation, the risk of rejection, and the delicate balance between immunosuppression and maintaining adequate immune function are all influenced by cortisol. Careful monitoring and management of cortisol levels become essential in ensuring the long-term success and viability of the transplanted organ.

Managing Cortisol Levels in Organ Failure and Transplantation:

Given the significant impact of cortisol on organ failure and transplantation, strategies for managing cortisol levels are essential. Here are some considerations:

Stress Reduction Techniques:

Incorporating stress reduction techniques such as mindfulness, meditation, deep breathing exercises, and relaxation therapies can help modulate cortisol levels and improve overall well-being.

Psychological Support:

Providing psychological support and counseling to individuals with organ failure and those undergoing transplantation can help mitigate stress, anxiety, and the associated cortisol response.

Medication Management:

Appropriate use of medications, including corticosteroids and immunosuppressants, is crucial in managing cortisol levels and maintaining immune system balance post-transplantation. Regular monitoring and adjustment of medication regimens are necessary to optimize outcomes.

Lifestyle Modifications:

Encouraging a healthy lifestyle, including regular exercise, a balanced diet, adequate sleep, and stress management, can help regulate cortisol levels and improve overall health in individuals with organ failure and those who have undergone transplantation.

So,

Cortisol plays a significant role in the body's response to organ failure and transplantation. Its impact on immune function, metabolic balance, and cardiovascular health underscores the importance of managing cortisol levels throughout the journey of organ transplantation. By recognizing the interplay between cortisol and organ failure, healthcare providers can develop comprehensive strategies to optimize patient outcomes and improve the success of transplantation. Continued research and advancements in cortisol management hold promise for enhancing the lives of individuals affected by organ failure and those embarking on the remarkable journey of transplantation.

So,

As we reach the final pages of this book, we reflect on the vast array of knowledge and insights we have gained about cortisol and its profound impact on our health and well-being. From its role in the stress response to its influence on various body systems and its connections to a myriad of diseases and conditions, cortisol has proven to be a remarkable hormone deserving of our attention and understanding.

Throughout these chapters, we have explored the intricate web of cortisol's effects on our bodies and minds. We have learned how cortisol affects our response to stress, shaping our ability to adapt and recover. We have witnessed its interactions with different body systems, from the immune system and cardiovascular system to the reproductive system and beyond. We have explored the role of cortisol in mental health, metabolism, bone health, and even the development and progression of chronic diseases.

One of the key takeaways from our journey is the delicate balance required in cortisol regulation. While cortisol is essential for our survival and well-being, excessive or prolonged elevation can have detrimental effects on our health. Recognizing this delicate balance empowers us to explore strategies for managing cortisol levels and optimizing our overall health and resilience.

We have explored various avenues for cortisol management, including lifestyle modifications, stress reduction techniques, medication management, and the importance of social support. By implementing these strategies, we can strive for a more harmonious cortisol response and foster a state of balance and well-being.

We hope that we have succeeded in making the intricacies of cortisol accessible to readers of all backgrounds. Whether you are a healthcare professional seeking deeper insights, a student eager to expand your knowledge, or an individual passionate about holistic well-being, we hope that this book has provided you with a comprehensive understanding of cortisol and its vital role in our lives.

As we conclude this enlightening journey, we invite you to carry the knowledge you have gained forward into your own life and the lives of others. Use this understanding of cortisol to enhance your own well-being, make informed choices, and support those around you in their pursuit of health and resilience.

Remember that cortisol is just one piece of the intricate puzzle that makes up our bodies and minds. By embracing a holistic approach to health, incorporating healthy habits, managing stress, nurturing social connections, and seeking professional guidance when needed, we can create a foundation of well-being that extends far beyond the realm of cortisol.

With this newfound understanding, we can embark on a journey of empowered health, armed with the knowledge to navigate the intricate interplay between cortisol and our overall well-being. Let us continue to explore, learn, and thrive as we embrace the transformative potential of understanding cortisol and its remarkable influence on our lives.

Thank you for accompanying us on this extraordinary voyage. May your journey be filled with health, resilience, and a profound appreciation for the wondrous workings of our bodies and minds.

___**Thanks**___ for going through all of the book chapters until the end!
Your review is ___**Valuable**___ to us as publishers.

Please consider leaving your _honest feedback_ on this book and help others benefit from it.

Made with the help of: chat.openai.com

www.ingramcontent.com/pod-product-compliance
Lightning Source LLC
Chambersburg PA
CBHW071218260726
48653CB00042B/1027